OXFORD ASSESS AND PROGRESS

Series Editors

Katharine Boursicot
Director, Health Professional Assessment Consultancy (HPAC)
Honorary Reader in Medical Education St George's,
University of London

David Sales
Consultant in Medical Assessment

OXFORD ASSESS AND PROGRESS
your prescription for exam success

Written by clinicians and educational experts, these unique guides present complete coverage for your exam revision, with illustrative material and tips to help you succeed in your medical exams.

Also available and forthcoming titles in the Oxford Assess and Progress series

Clinical Medicine, Second Edition
Alex Liakos and Martin Hill

Clinical Surgery
Neil Borley, Frank Smith, Paul McGovern, Bernadette Pereira, and Oliver Old

Emergency Medicine
Pawan Gupta

Medical Sciences
Jade Chow and John Patterson

Psychiatry
Gil Myers and Melissa Gardner

Situational Judgement Test, Third Edition
David Metcalfe and Harveer Dev

OXFORD ASSESS AND PROGRESS

Clinical Specialties

Third Edition

Edited by

Luci Etheridge

Consultant Paediatrician and Honorary Senior Lecturer in Clinical Education, St George's University Hospitals NHS Foundation Trust and St George's, University of London

Alex Bonner

Consultant Anaesthetist, Lancashire Teaching Hospitals NHS Foundation Trust

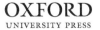

OXFORD
UNIVERSITY PRESS

OXFORD
UNIVERSITY PRESS

Great Clarendon Street, Oxford, OX2 6DP,
United Kingdom

Oxford University Press is a department of the University of Oxford.
It furthers the University's objective of excellence in research, scholarship,
and education by publishing worldwide. Oxford is a registered trade mark of
Oxford University Press in the UK and in certain other countries

First Edition published in 2010
Second Edition published in 2013
Third Edition published in 2018

Impression: 2

Published in the United States of America by Oxford University Press
198 Madison Avenue, New York, NY 10016, United States of America

British Library Cataloguing in Publication Data

Data available

Library of Congress Control Number: 201796221

ISBN 978–0–19–880290–7

Printed and bound in Great Britain by
Ashford Colour Press Ltd.

Series editor preface

The Oxford Assess and Progress series is a groundbreaking development in the extensive area of self-assessment texts available for medical students. The questions were specifically commissioned for the series, written by practising clinicians, extensively peer-reviewed by students and their teachers, and quality-assured to ensure that the material is up-to-date, accurate, and in line with modern testing formats.

The series has a number of unique features and is designed to be as much a formative learning resource as a self-assessment one. The questions are constructed to test the same clinical problem-solving skills that we use as practising clinicians, rather than only to test theoretical knowledge. These skills include:

- gathering and using data required for clinical judgement
- choosing the appropriate examination and investigations, and interpretation of the findings
- applying knowledge
- demonstrating diagnostic skills
- ability to evaluate undifferentiated material
- ability to prioritize
- making decisions and demonstrating a structured approach to decision-making.

Each question is bedded in reality and is typically presented as a clinical scenario, the content of which has been chosen to reflect the common and important conditions that most doctors are likely to encounter both during their training and in exams! The aim of the series is to build the reader's confidence in recognizing important symptoms and signs and suggesting the most appropriate investigations and management, and in so doing to aid the development of a clear approach to patient management which can be transferred to the wards.

The content of the series has deliberately been pinned to the relevant *Oxford Handbook* but, in addition, has been guided by a blueprint which reflects the themes identified in *Tomorrow's Doctors* and *Good Medical Practice* to include novel areas such as history taking, recognition of signs (including red flags), and professionalism.

Particular attention has been paid to giving learning points and constructive feedback on each question, using clear fact- or evidence-based explanations as to why the correct response is right and why the incorrect responses are less appropriate. The question editorials are clearly referenced to the relevant sections of the accompanying *Oxford Handbook* and/or more widely to medical literature or guidelines. They are designed to guide and motivate the reader, being multi-purpose in nature and covering, for example, exam technique, approaches to difficult subjects, and links between subjects.

Another unique aspect of the series is the element of competency progression from being a relatively inexperienced student to being a more experienced junior doctor. We have suggested the following four degrees of difficulty to reflect the level of training, so that the reader can monitor their own progress over time:

- graduate should know ★
- graduate nice to know ★★
- foundation doctor should know ★★★
- foundation doctor nice to know ★★★★

We advise the reader to attempt the questions in blocks as a way of testing their knowledge in a clinical context. The series can be treated as a dress rehearsal for life on the ward by using the material to hone clinical acumen and build confidence by encouraging a clear, consistent, and rational approach, proficiency in recognizing and evaluating symptoms and signs, making a rational differential diagnosis, and suggesting appropriate investigations and management.

Adopting such an approach can aid not only success in examinations, which really are designed to confirm learning, but also—more importantly—being a good doctor. In this way, we can deliver high-quality and safe patient care by recognizing, understanding, and treating common problems, but at the same time remaining alert to the possibility of less likely, but potentially catastrophic, conditions.

David Sales and Kathy Boursicot
Series Editors

A note on single best answer questions

Single best answer questions are currently the format of choice being widely used by most undergraduate and postgraduate knowledge tests, and therefore all of the assessment questions in this book follow this format.

Single best answer questions have many advantages over other machine-markable formats, such as extended matching questions (EMQs), notably the breadth of sampling or content coverage that they afford.

Briefly, the single best answer or 'best of five' question presents a problem, usually a clinical scenario, before presenting the question itself and a list of five options. These consist of one correct answer and four incorrect options or 'distractors', from which the reader has to choose a response.

All of the questions in this book, which are typically based on an evaluation of symptoms, signs, or results of investigations, either as single entities or in combination, are designed to test *reasoning* skills, rather than straightforward recall of facts, and utilize cognitive processes similar to those used in clinical practice.

The peer-reviewed questions are written and edited in accordance with contemporary best assessment practice, and their content has been guided by a blueprint pinned to all areas of *Good Medical Practice*, which ensures comprehensive coverage.

The answers and their rationales are evidence-based and have been reviewed to ensure that they are absolutely correct. Incorrect options are selected as being plausible, and indeed they may appear correct to the less knowledgeable reader. When answering questions, the reader may wish to use the 'cover' test in which they read the scenario and the question but cover the options.

Kathy Boursicot and David Sales
Series Editors

Editor preface to the third edition

During the journey through medical school as a student, you experience medicine in a range of settings, from the rural general practice to the inner-city teaching hospital. You encounter doctors working in a wide range of specialties, many of which will be appealing future career choices and many of which will seem daunting. Specialty attachments may be the first time that you encounter people with mental illness, or children, or pregnant women. Trying to absorb all of these new experiences while also continuing to work towards final examinations can seem like a roller-coaster ride to some!

In partnership with the well-established *Oxford Handbook of Clinical Specialties*, the *Oxford Assess and Progress: Clinical Specialties* volume seeks to tie together the clinical specialties and to provide a grounding in knowledge that may get pushed to the back burner when medicine and surgery have to be revised. This third edition has been produced in line with the new edition of the *Oxford Handbook of Clinical Specialties* and builds on the success of the first and second books, bringing you questions on the latest hot topics, current issues, and core material. In line with the new edition of *Oxford Handbook of Clinical Specialties*, this latest edition has a chapter on eponymous syndromes. While students may not encounter many of these rare or unusual conditions during the early years of their practice, they constitute useful material for examination questions at all stages. There are also enhanced chapters on obstetrics, gynaecology, orthopaedics, and trauma, and a new chapter on pre-hospital care. This ensures the full spectrum of specialty practice is considered and covered.

The questions in each chapter have been written by experienced doctors working within the specialty, who are familiar with the common presentations, pathologies, and dilemmas that are encountered. Their knowledge of teaching medical students about their specialty, often within the confines of very short attachments, has been transferred to these pages. All of the questions map on to medical school curricula and are rooted in real-life clinical encounters. The grading system allows you to judge for yourself which knowledge is core and which might require some further reading. We have added many new guidelines and key websites to guide this reading, and we hope that you will find these useful. The strong focus on clinical experiences also allows you to look forward to, and prepare for, your time as a foundation doctor.

We hope that, as a result of working through these questions, your interest in, and appreciation and understanding of, the different clinical specialties will grow, and you will have a useful tool for judging your own learning needs.

Luci Etheridge and Alex Bonner

Acknowledgements

The editors would like to thank all of the contributors from all editions for their hard work in combining their specialist knowledge with clinical experience to provide this resource of stimulating, realistic questions with considered explanations. Sadly, one of our much valued contributors Dr Gill McGauley passed away in 2016. Gill was a well-known and respected psychiatrist and educationalist, and we are grateful to her for being one of the original contributors to this Series. Thank you also to all of the reviewers—students and specialists—for your much valued feedback. We hope that we have managed to address your suggestions in this new edition. Finally, Luci would like to thank her ever patient children, who are a constant source of inspiration and joy. Alex and his wife Amy are now also joined by two children Frederick and Arthur since the second edition.

Contents

About the editors

Volume editors

Luci Etheridge is a Consultant Paediatrician and Honorary Senior Lecturer in Clinical Education at St George's University Hospitals NHS Foundation Trust in London. She previously worked for four years with UCL Medical School and was involved with the development of Fitness to Practise assessments for the General Medical Council and item writing for the Professional and Linguistics Assessments Board Part 1 and the Royal College of Paediatrics and Child Health. She has a doctorate in education from the Institute of Education, University of London, and plays an active role in undergraduate and postgraduate education, regionally and nationally, in the UK.

Alex Bonner is a Consultant Anaesthetist at Lancashire Teaching Hospitals NHS Foundation Trust, with subspecialty interests in vascular anaesthesia and medical education. He is regularly involved in the teaching of medical students, foundation doctors, and anaesthetic trainees who are preparing for their FRCA examinations. He is an instructor for Adult and Paediatric Advanced Life Support courses and has experience of practising anaesthesia and teaching in sub-Saharan Africa. He has also contributed to the development of Fitness to Practise assessments for the General Medical Council.

Series editors

Katharine Boursicot BSc MBBS MRCOG MAHPE NTF SFHEA FRSM is a consultant in health professions education, with special expertise in assessment. Previously, she was Head of Assessment at St George's, University of London, Barts and The London School of Medicine and Dentistry, and Associate Dean for Assessment at Cambridge University School of Clinical Medicine. She is a consultant on assessment to several UK medical schools, medical Royal Colleges, and international institutions, as well as an assessment advisor to the General Medical Council.

David Sales is a general practitioner by training who has been involved in medical assessment for over 20 years, having previously been convenor of the MRCGP knowledge test. He has run item-writing workshops for a number of undergraduate medical schools and medical Royal Colleges, and internationally. He currently chairs the Professional and Linguistic Assessments Board Part 1 panel for the General Medical Council and is their consultant on Fitness to Practise knowledge testing.

Previous edition contributors

Erica Allason-Jones
NHS consultant in Genitourinary Medicine, Mortimer Market Centre (Camden PCT), London, UK

Dinesh Bhugra
Professor of Mental Health and Cultural Diversity at the Institute of Psychiatry, King's College, London, and Honorary Consultant, Maudsley Hospital, London, UK

Jennifer Birch
Consultant in Neonatal Medicine, Luton and Dunstable NHS Foundation Hospital Trust, Luton, UK

Alex Bonner
Specialist Trainee in Anaesthesia and Critical Care, North West Deanery, UK

Ruth Brown
Consultant in Emergency Medicine, St Mary's Hospital, Imperial College NHS Trust, and Honorary Senior Lecturer, Imperial College London, UK

Will Coppola
Clinical Lecturer and Sub-Dean E-learning, UCL Medical School, London, UK, and salaried General Practitioner

Jonathan Darling
Senior Lecturer in Paediatrics and Child Health, University of Leeds, and Honorary Consultant Paediatrician, Leeds Teaching Hospitals NHS Trust, Leeds, UK

Nev Davies
Consultant in Trauma and Orthopaedics, Royal Berkshire Hospital, Reading, UK

James Dawson
Registrar in Anaesthesia and Intensive Care, Trent Region, UK

Philippa Edwards
Salaried General Practitioner, Portsmouth, UK

Luci Etheridge
Consultant Paediatrician and Senior Fellow in Clinical Leadership, Barking, Havering and Redbridge University Hospitals NHS Trust, London, UK

Kamila Hawthorne
General Practice Principal in Cardiff, and Sub Dean for Assessment, School of Medicine, Cardiff University, Cardiff, UK

Kevin Hayes
Senior Lecturer and Consultant in Obstetrics and Gynaecology, St George's Hospital, London, UK

Virginia Hubbard
Consultant Dermatologist, Homerton University Hospital, and Clinical Senior Lecturer, Barts and the London School of Medicine and Dentistry, UK

Vikram Jha
Senior Lecturer in Medical Education, Leeds Institute of Medical Education, University of Leeds, and Honorary Consultant Obstetrician, Bradford Teaching Hospitals NHS Trust, UK

Matthew Mathai
Consultant Paediatrician,
Bradford Royal Infirmary, and
Honorary Lecturer in Paediatrics
and Child Health, University of
Leeds, UK

Gill McGauley
Reader in Forensic
Psychotherapy, St George's
University of London, and
Consultant in Forensic
Psychotherapy, Broadmoor
Hospital, West London Mental
Health NHS Trust, UK

Isabel McMullen
Specialty Registrar in Psychiatry,
South London and Maudsley NHS
Foundation Trust, UK

Zeryab Setna
Research Fellow in Medical
Education, Leeds Institute of
Medical Education, University of
Leeds, Leeds, UK

Venki Sundaram
Specialty Registrar in
Ophthalmology, London
Deanery, London, UK

Philippa Tostevin
Senior Lecturer in Surgical
Education, St George's University
of London, and Honorary
Consultant Otolaryngologist,
St George's Hospital, London, UK

Contributors

Alex Bonner
Consultant Anaesthetist,
Lancashire Teaching Hospitals
NHS Foundation Trust

Nev Davies
Consultant in Trauma &
Orthopaedics, Royal Berkshire
Hospital, Reading, UK

Philippa Edwards
General Practice, Locum GP in
Barnet, UK

Luci Etheridge
Consultant Paediatrician and
Honorary Senior Lecturer in
Clinical Education, St George's
University Hospitals NHS
Foundation Trust and
St George's University of
London, London, UK

Oliver Harrison
Consultant Anaesthetist,
Department of Anaesthesia,
Royal Preston Hospital and North
West Air Ambulance

Kevin Hayes
Consultant Gynaecologist,
St George's University Hospital,
London, UK and Senior Lecturer
in Obstetrics and Gynaecology,
St George's, University of
London, UK

Isabel McMullen
Consultant Liaison Psychiatrist,
Department of Psychological
Medicine, South London and
Maudsley NHS Foundation Trust,
King's College Hospital, UK

Catherine Roberts
Consultant in Emergency
Medicine, Emergency Medicine
Department, Royal Preston
Hospital, Lancashire Teaching
Hospitals NHS Foundation
Trust, UK

Zeryab Setna
Consultant Obstetrician, Lady
Dufferin Hospital, Karachi,
Pakistan

Gemma Simcox
Salaried General Practitioner with
Special Interest in Dermatology,
West Yorkshire, UK

Venki Sundaram
Consultant Ophthalmologist,
Department of Ophthalmology,
Luton and Dunstable NHS
University Hospital, UK

Philippa Tostevin
Course Director MBBS, Reader
in Surgical Education, St George's
University of London; Consultant
ENT Surgeon, St Georges NHS
Foundation Trust, London, UK

Anuhya Vusirikala
Core Surgical Trainee, Oxford
Deanery, UK

Normal and average values

Biochemistry: reference intervals

All laboratory discourse is probabilistic. Drugs may interfere with any chemical method; as these effects may be method-dependent, it is difficult for us to be aware of all of the possibilities. If in doubt, discuss the issue with the laboratory.

Substance	Specimen	Normal value
Adrenocorticotrophic hormone	P	<80 ng/L
Alanine aminotransferase	P	5–35 IU/L
Albumin	P†	35–50 g/L
Aldosterone	P*	100–500 pmol/L
Alkaline phosphatase	P†	30–150 IU/L (adults)
α-fetoprotein	S	<10 kU/L
α-amylase	P	0–180 Somogyi units/dL
Angiotensin II	P*	5–35 pmol/L
Antidiuretic hormone	P	0.9–4.6 pmol/L
Aspartate transaminase	P	5–35 IU/L
β-HCG	S	M: <10 mIU/mL; F (non-pregnant): <25 mIU/mL; F (4 weeks pregnant): >1000 mIU/mL
Bicarbonate	P†	24–30 mmol/L
Bilirubin	P	3–17 μmol/L (0.25–1.5 mg/100 mL)
Calcitonin	P	<0.1 micrograms/L
Calcium (ionized)	P	1.0–1.25 mmol/L
Calcium (total)	P†	2.12–2.65 mmol/L
Chloride	P	95–105 mmol/L
Cholesterol‡	P	3.9–7.8 mmol/L
VLDL	P	0.128–0.645 mmol/L
LDL	P	1.55–4.4 mmol/L
HDL	P	0.9–1.93 mmol/L

Substance	Specimen	Normal value
Cortisol	P	a.m.: 450–700 nmol/L; midnight: 80–280 nmol/L
C-reactive protein (CRP)	S	<10 mg/L
Creatine kinase	P	M: 25–195 IU/L; F: 25–170 IU/L
Creatinine (related to lean body mass)	P†	70–≤150 µmol/L
CSF glucose	CSF	>2/3 of blood range
CSF protein	CSF	<40 mg/dL
CSF white cells	CSF	<5/mm³
Ferritin	P	12–200 micrograms/L
Folate	S	2.1 micrograms/L
Follicle-stimulating hormone (FSH)	P/S	Luteal: 2–8 U/L Ovulatory peak: 8–15 U/L Follicular phase, and M: 0.5–5 U/L Post-menopausal: >30 U/L
Gamma-glutamyl transpeptidase	P	M: 11–51 IU/L; F: 7–33 IU/L
Glucose (fasting)	P	3.5–5 mmol/L
Glycated (glycosylated) haemoglobin	B	<48 mmol/mol
Growth hormone	P	< 20 mU/L
Iron	S	M: 14–31 µmol/L; F: 11–30 µmol/L
Lactate dehydrogenase (LDH)	P	70–250 IU/L
Lead	B	<1.8 mmol/L
Luteinizing hormone	P/S	Pre-menopausal: 3–13 U/L Follicular: 3–12 U/L Ovulatory peak: 20–80 U/L Luteal: 3–16 U/L Post-menopausal: >30 U/L
Magnesium	P	0.75–1.05 mmol/L
Osmolality	P	278–305 mOsmol/kg
Parathyroid hormone (PTH)	P	<0.8–8.5 pmol/L
Phosphate (inorganic)	P	0.8–1.45 mmol/L
Potassium	P	3.5–5.0 mmol/L
Prolactin	P	M: <450 U/L; F: <600 U/L
Prostate-specific antigen	P	0–4 ng/mL
Protein (total)	P	60–80 g/L

Substance	Specimen	Normal value
Red cell folate	B	0.36–1.44 µmol/L (160–640 micrograms/L)
Renin (erect/recumbent)	P*	2.8–4.5/1.1–2.7 pmol/mL/hour
Sodium	P†	135–145 mmol/L
Thyroid-binding globulin (TBG)	P	7–17 mg/L
Thyroid-stimulating hormone (TSH) (normal range widens with age)	P	0.5–5.7 mU/L
Thyroxine (T4)	P	70–140 nmol/L
Thyroxine (free)	P	9–22 pmol/L
Total iron-binding capacity	S	54–75 µmol/L
Triglyceride	P	0.55–1.90 mmol/L
Tri-iodothyronine	P	1.2–3.0 nmol/L
Urea	P†	2.5–6.7 mmol/L
Urate	P†	M: 210–480 µmol/L; F: 150–390 µmol/L
Vitamin B$_{12}$	S	0.13–0.68 nmol/L (<150 ng/L)

* The sample requires special handling. Contact the laboratory.
† Range is significantly different in pregnancy (see table in later text).
‡ Desired upper limit of cholesterol level would be <5 mmol/L.
Abbreviations: P, plasma (heparin bottle); S, serum (clotted; no anticoagulant); B, whole blood (edetic acid (EDTA) bottle); CSF, cerebrospinal fluid specimen; IU, international unit; M, males; F, females; HDL, high-density lipoprotein; LDL, low-density lipoprotein; VLDL, very-low-density lipoprotein.

Arterial blood gases

pH	7.35–7.45
P$_a$CO$_2$	4.7–6.0 kPa
P$_a$O$_2$	<10.6 kPa
Base excess	± 2 mmol/L

Note: 7.6 mmHg = 1 kPa (atmospheric pressure ≈ 100 kPa).

Haematology: reference intervals

Measurement	Reference interval
White cell count (WCC)	$4.0–11.0 \times 10^9$/L
Red cell count	M: $4.5–6.5 \times 10^{12}$/L; F: $3.9–5.6 \times 10^{12}$/L
Haemoglobin	M: 13.5–18.0 g/dL; F: 11.5–16.0 g/dL
Packed red cell volume (PCV) or haematocrit	M: 0.4–0.54 l/L; F: 0.37–0.47 l/L
Mean cell volume (MCV)	76–96 fL
Mean cell haemoglobin (MCH)	27–32 pg
Mean cell haemoglobin concentration (MCHC)	30–36 g/dL
Neutrophil count	$2.0–7.5 \times 10^9$/L; 40–75% WCC
Lymphocyte count	$1.3–3.5 \times 10^9$/L; 20–45% WCC
Eosinophil count	$0.04–0.44 \times 10^9$/L; 1–6% WCC
Basophil count	$0.0–0.1 \times 10^9$/L; 0–1% WCC
Monocyte count	$0.2–0.8 \times 10^9$/L; 2–10% WCC
Platelet count	$150–400 \times 10^9$/L
Reticulocyte count	$25–100 \times 10^9$/L; 0.8–2.0%
Erythrocyte sedimentation rate	<20 mm/hour (but depends on age; see OHCM 10th edn, p. 372)
Activated partial thromboplastin time (VIII, IX, XI, XII)	35–45 seconds
Prothrombin time	10–14 seconds

International normalized ratio (INR)	Clinical state (see OHCM 10th edn, p. 351)
2.0–3.0	Treatment of deep vein thrombosis (DVT), pulmonary emboli (treat for 3–6 months)
2.5–3.5	Embolism prophylaxis in atrial fibrillation (see OHCM 10th edn, p. 351)
3.0–4.5	Recurrent DVT and pulmonary embolism; arterial disease, including myocardial infarction; arterial grafts; cardiac prosthetic valves (if caged ball, aim for 4–4.9) and grafts

Plasma chemistry in pregnancy

	Non-pregnant		Trimester 1		Trimester 2		Trimester 3	
Centile	2.5	97.5	2.5	97.5	2.5	97.5	2.5	97.5
Na$^+$ (mmol/L)	138	146	135	141	132	140	133	141
Ca^{2+} (mmol/L)	2	2.6	2.3	2.5	2.2	2.2	2.2	2.5
Corrected*	2.3	2.6	2.25	2.57	2.3	2.5	2.3	2.59
Albumin (g/L)	44	50	39	49	36	44	33	41
Free T$_4$ (pmol/L)	9	23	10	24	9	19	7	17
Free T$_3$ (pmol/L)	4	9	4	8	4	7	3	5
TSH	0	4	0	1.6	1	1.8	7	7.3

* Calcium corrected for plasma albumin (see OHCM 10th edn, p. 676).

Other plasma reference intervals (not analysed by trimester)

	Non-pregnant	Pregnant
Alkaline phosphatase (IU/L)	3–300	Up to 450*
Bicarbonate (mmol/L)	24–30	20–25
Creatinine (μmol/L)	70–150	24–68
Urea (mmol/L)	2.5–6.7	2–4.2
Urate (μmol/L)	150–390	100–270

* Occasionally very much higher in apparently normal pregnancies.

- C-reactive protein levels do not change much during pregnancy.
- TSH levels may be low in the first half of a normal pregnancy (suppressed by HCG). For other thyroid changes, see earlier text and OHCS 10th edn, p. 25.
- Protein S levels fall during pregnancy, so protein S deficiency is difficult to diagnose.
- Activated protein C (APC) resistance is found in 40% of pregnancies, so special tests are required when looking for this. Genotyping for factor V Leiden and prothrombin G20210A is unaffected by pregnancy.

Paediatric reference intervals

Laboratories vary, so it is important to consult your own.

	Specimen	Normal value
Biochemistry (1 mmol = 1 mEq/L)		
Albumin	P	36–48 g/dL
Alkaline phosphatase	P	Depends on age*
α1-antitrypsin	P	1.3–3.4 g/dL
Ammonium	P	2–25 µmol/L; 3–35 micrograms/dL
Amylase	P	70–300 U/L
Aspartate aminotransferase	P	<40 U/L
Bilirubin	P	2–16 µmol/L; 0.1–0.8 mg/dL
Bicarbonate	P	21–25 mmol/L
Calcium	P	2.25–2.75 mmol/L; 9–11 mg/dL
Neonates		1.72–2.47 mmol/L; 6.9–9.9 mg/dL
Chloride	P	98–105 mmol/L
Cholesterol	P, F	≤5.7 mmol/L; 100–200 mg/dL
Creatine kinase	P	<80 U/L
Creatinine	P	25–115 µmol/L; 0.3–1.3 mg/dL
Glucose	F	2.5–5.3 mmol/L; 45–95 mg/dL (lower in newborn; fluoride tube)
IgA	S	0.8–4.5 g/L (low at birth, rising to adult level slowly)
IgG	S	5–18 g/L (high at birth, then falls, and finally rises slowly to adult level)
IgM	S	0.2–2.0 g/L (low at birth, rising to adult level by 1 year)
IgE	S	<500 U/mL
Iron	S	9–36 µmol/L; 50–200 micrograms/dL
Lead	EDTA	<1.75 µmol/L; <36 micrograms/dL
Mg²⁺	P	0.6–1.0 mmol/L
Osmolality	P	275–295 mosmol/L
Phenylalanine	P	0.04–0.21 mmol/L
Potassium (mean)	P	3.5–5.5 mmol/L
Protein	P	63–81 g/L; 6.3–8.1 g/dL
Sodium	P	136–145 mmol/L
Transferrin	S	2.5–4.5 g/L

	Specimen	Normal value
Triglycerides	F, S	0.34–1.92 mmol/L (30–170 mg/dL)
Urate	P	0.12–0.36 mmol/L; 2–6 mg/dL
Urea	P	2.5–6.6 mmol/L; 15–40 mg/dL
Gamma-glutamyl transferase	P	<20 U/L
Hormones: a guide (consult laboratory)		
Cortisol	P	9 a.m.: 200–700 nmol/L; midnight: <140 nmol/L (mean)
Dehydroepiandrosterone sulfate	P	Days 5–11 of life: 0.8–2.8 μmol/L (range); 5–11 years: 0.1–3.6 μmol/L
17α-hydroxyprogesterone	P	Days 5–11 of life: 1.6–7.5 nmol/L (range); 4–11 years: 0.4–4.2 nmol/L
T$_4$	P	60–135 nmol/L (not neonates)
TSH	P	<5 mU/L (higher on days 1–4)

* Alkaline phosphatase (U/L): 0–0.5 years: 150–600; 0.5–2 years: 250–1000; 2–5 years: 250–850; 6–7 years: 250–1000; 8–9 years: 250–750; 10–11 years: G = 259–950, B = ≤730; 12–13 years: G = 200–750, B = ≤785; 14–15 years: G = 170–460, B = 170–970; 16–17 years: G = 75–270, B = 125–720; <18 years: G = 60–250, B = 50–200.
Abbreviations: B, boys; EDTA, edetic acid; F, fasting; G, girls; P, plasma; S, serum.

Haematology (mean ± ~1 standard deviation; range × 10⁹/L (median in parentheses))

	Hb (g/dL)	MCV (fL)	MCHC (%)	Reticulocyte count (%)	White cell count	Neutrophil count	Eosinophil count	Lymphocyte count	Monocyte count
Days									
1	19.0 ± 2	119 ± 9	31.6 ± 2	3.2 ± 1	9–30	6–26 (11)	0.02–0.8	2–11	0.4–3.1
4	18.6 ± 2	114 ± 7	32.6 ± 2	1.8 ± 1	9–40				
5	17.6 ± 1	114 ± 9	30.9 ± 2	1.2 ± 0.2					
Weeks									
1–2	17.3 ± 2	112 ± 19	32.1 ± 3	0.5 ± 0.03	5–21	1.5–10 (5)	0.07–0.1	2–17	0.3–2.7
2–3	15.6 ± 3	111 ± 8	33.9 ± 2	0.8 ± 0.6	6–15	1–9.5 (4)	0.07–0.1	2–17	0.2–2.4
4–5	12.7 ± 2	101 ± 8	34.9 ± 2	0.9 ± 0.8	6–15	(4)		(6)	
6–7	12.0 ± 2	105 ± 12	33.8 ± 2	1.2 ± 0.7	6–15	(4)		(6)	
8–9	10.7 ± 1	93 ± 12	34.1 ± 2	1.8 ± 1	6–15	(4)		(6)	
Months (all the following Hb values are medians/lower limit for normal)									
3	11.5/9	88/88			6–15	(3)		(6)	
6	11.5/9	77/70			6–15	(3)		(6)	
12	11.5/9	78/72			6–15	(3)		(6)	
Years									
2	11.5/9	78/74			6–15	(3)		(5)	
4	12.2/10	80/75			6–15	(4)		(4)	
6	13/10.4	82/75			5–15	(4.2)		(3.8)	

12	13.8/11	83/76			4–13	(4.9)		(3.1)	
14B	14.2/12	84/77			4–13	(5)		(3)	
14G	14/11.5								
16B	14.8/12	85/78	30–36	0.8–2	4–13	2–7.5 (5)	0.04–0.4	1.3–3.5	0.2–0.8
16G	14/11.5								
18B	15/13								

Note:
Basophil range: 0–0.1 × 10⁹/L; vitamin B_{12} (serum): ≥150 ng/L.
Red cell folate (EDTA): 100–640 ng/mL.
Platelet counts do not vary with age: 150–400 × 10⁹/L.
Abbreviations: B, boys; G, girls.

Abbreviations

ABC	Airway, breathing, and circulation
ABCDE	Airway, breathing, circulation, disability, and exposure
ADHD	Attention-deficit/hyperactivity disorder
ALS	Advanced Life Support
ASA	American Society of Anesthesiologists
ATLS	Advanced Trauma Life Support
AUDIT	Alcohol Use Disorders Identification Test
BCC	Basal cell carcinoma
BD	Twice daily
BMI	Body mass index
BNF	*British National Formulary*
BP	Blood pressure
bpm	Beats per minute
BPPV	Benign paroxysmal positional vertigo
BSA	Body surface area
C	Celsius
CD4+	Cluster of differentiation 4
CHC	Combined hormonal contraceptive
CIN	Cervical intraepithelial neoplasia
CKD	Chronic kidney disease
cm	Centimetre
CNS	Central nervous system
CO	Carbon monoxide
CO_2	Carbon dioxide
COPD	Chronic obstructive pulmonary disease
CPAP	Continuous positive airway pressure
CPR	Cardiopulmonary resuscitation
CRP	C-reactive protein
CSF	Cerebrospinal fluid
CT	Computed tomography
CTG	Cardiotocography
CVD	Cardiovascular disease
CVP	Central venous pressure
dB	Decibel

DDH	Developmental dysplasia of the hip
DEXA	Dual-energy X-ray absorptiometry
DKA	Diabetic ketoacidosis
dL	Decilitre
DMSA	Dimercaptosuccinic acid
DNA	Deoxyribonucleic acid
DVLA	Driver and Vehicle Licensing Agency
EAS	External anal sphincter
ECG	Electrocardiogram
ECV	External cephalic version
EEG	Electroencephalogram
ENT	Ear, nose, and throat
ERCP	Endoscopic retrograde cholangiopancreatography
ESR	Erythrocyte sedimentation rate
FBC	Full blood count
fL	Fluid ounce
FSH	Follicle-stimulating hormone
FTA-ABS	Fluorescent treponemal antibody absorption test
FU	Fluorouracil
g	Gram
G	Gauge
GABA	Gamma-aminobutyric acid
GAG	Glycosaminoglycan
GCS	Glasgow Coma Scale
GFR	Glomerular filtration rate
GGT	Gamma-glutamyl transpeptidase
GI	Gastrointestinal
GMC	General Medical Council
GP	General practitioner
HART	Hazardous Area Response Team
Hb	Haemoglobin
HBcAb	Hepatitis B virus core antibody
HBeAg	Hepatitis B virus e antigen
HBsAb	Hepatitis B virus surface antibody
HBsAg	Hepatitis B virus surface antigen
HBV	Hepatitis B virus
HCG	Human chorionic gonadotrophin
HCO_3	Bicarbonate
Hg	Mercury

HIV	Human immunodeficiency virus
HPV	Human papillomavirus
HRT	Hormone replacement therapy
IAS	Internal anal sphincter
Ig	Immunoglobulin
IM	Intramuscular
INR	International normalized ratio
IQ	Intelligence quotient
IU	International unit
IUD	Intrauterine device
IUS	Intrauterine system
IV	Intravenous
IVF	*In-vitro* fertilization
kg	Kilogram
kPa	Kilopascal
KTD	Kendrick traction device
kU	Kilo-unit
L	Litre
LFT	Liver function test
LH	Luteinizing hormone
LPA	Lasting Power of Attorney
m	Metre
MAOI	Monoamine oxidase inhibitor
MAST	Military anti-shock trousers
MCHC	Mean corpuscular haemoglobin concentration
MCNS	Minimal change nephrotic syndrome
MCV	Mean corpuscular volume
mEq	Milli-equivalent
MEWS	Modified Early Warning Score
mg	Milligram
MI	Myocardial infarction
min	Minute
mIU	Milli-international unit
mL	Millilitre
mm	Millimetre
mmol	Millimole
MMSE	Mini-Mental State Examination
mol	Mole
mosmol	Milliosmole

mph	Miles per hour
MPS	mucopolysaccharidosis
MRI	Magnetic resonance imaging
mU	Milli-unit
NEB	By nebulizer
ng	Nanogram
NICE	National Institute for Health and Care Excellence
NIPT	Non-invasive prenatal testing
NIV	Non-invasive ventilation
nmol	Nanomole
NSAID	Non-steroidal anti-inflammatory drug
O_2	Oxygen
OAV	oculo-auriculo-vertebral
OD	Once daily
OHCM	*Oxford Handbook of Clinical Medicine*
OHCS	*Oxford Handbook of Clinical Specialties*
OP	Occiput posterior
ORT	Oral rehydration therapy
P_aCO_2	Partial pressure of carbon dioxide in arterial blood
P_aO_2	Partial pressure of oxygen in arterial blood
PCI	Percutaneous coronary intervention
pCO_2	Partial pressure of carbon dioxide
PCOS	Polycystic ovary syndrome
PCP	*Pneumocystis carinii* pneumonia
PEP	Post-exposure prophylaxis
pg	Picogram
PHEM	Pre-hospital emergency medicine
pmol	Picomole
PO	*Per os* (by mouth)
pO_2	Partial pressure of oxygen
RPR	Rapid plasma reagin
SCC	Squamous cell carcinoma
SGLT2	sodium–glucose co-transporter-2
SLE	Systemic lupus erythematosus
SSRI	Selective serotonin reuptake inhibitor
TB	Tuberculosis
TDS	Three times daily
TENS	Transcutaneous electrical nerve stimulation
THR	Total hip replacement

TIA	Transient ischaemic attack
TPPA	*Treponema pallidum* particle agglutination
TURP	Transurethral resection of the prostate
U	Unit
UK	United Kingdom
UTI	Urinary tract infection
VBAC	Vaginal birth after Caesarean section
VDRL	Venereal Disease Research Laboratory
VF	Ventricular fibrillation
VT	Ventricular tachycardia
WHO	World Health Organization
ZIG	Zoster immunoglobulin

How to use this book

Oxford Assess and Progress: Clinical Specialties has been carefully designed to ensure you get the most out of your revision and are prepared for your exams. Here is a brief guide to some of the features and learning tools.

Organization of content

Chapter editorials will help you unpick tricky subjects, and when it is late at night and you need something to remind you why you are doing this, you will find words of encouragement!

Answers can be found at the end of each chapter, in order.

How to read an answer

Unlike other revision guides on the market, this one is crammed full of feedback, so you should understand exactly why each answer is correct, and gain an insight into the common pitfalls. With every answer, there is an explanation of why that particular choice is the most appropriate. For some questions, there is additional explanation of why the distracters are less suitable. Where relevant, you will also be directed to sources of further information such as the *Oxford Handbook of Clinical Specialties*, websites, and journal articles.

→ http://www.bmj.com/cgi/content/full/334/7583/35

Progression points

The questions in every chapter are ordered by level of difficulty and competence, indicated by the following symbols:

★   *Graduate 'should know'*—you should be aiming to get most of these correct.

★★   *Graduate 'nice to know'*—these are a bit tougher but not above your capabilities.

★★★   *Foundation doctor 'should know'*—these will really test your understanding.

★★★★   *Foundation doctor 'nice to know'*—give these a go when you are ready to challenge yourself.

Oxford Handbook of Clinical Specialties

The OHCS page references are given with the answers to some questions (e.g. OHCS 10th edn → p. 340). Please note that this reference is the **tenth edition** of the OHCS, and that subsequent or previous editions are unlikely to have the same material in exactly the same place.

Chapter 1

Obstetrics

Zeryab Setna

This chapter will be of interest and help to all those studying the health-care of women. Obstetrics, like all fields of medicine, continues to evolve at a rapid pace, and keeping up-to-date with the latest literature, guidelines and protocols can be a daunting task. In the following questions we have tried to encompass all of the important areas of this subject.

Pregnancy can be a joyful experience for both the mother and her family. However, it can occasionally be associated with complications, resulting in severe short- and long-term harm to both the mother and her baby. This chapter covers the most important aspects of pregnancy and its commonly associated problems, drawing on important guidelines to highlight the core knowledge and skill practitioners in the field are expected to have.

QUESTIONS

1. An 18-year-old woman who is 34 weeks pregnant has abdominal pain and moderate fresh vaginal bleeding. The symphysio-fundal height measures 41 cm and the uterus feels tense and tender. The patient's pulse rate is 98 bpm and her blood pressure is 90/50 mmHg. Which is the single most likely diagnosis? ★

A Cervical ectropion

B Placental abruption

C Placenta praevia

D Pre-term labour

E Vasa praevia

2. A 22-year-old woman comes to the antenatal booking clinic at 12 weeks' gestation. Which is the single most appropriate group of booking investigations? ★

A Full blood count, blood group and hepatitis C serology

B Full blood count, blood group and Venereal Disease Research Laboratory (VDRL) test

C Full blood count, thalassaemia screen and thyroid function test

D Full blood count, thalassaemia screen and urea and electrolytes

E Full blood count, thyroid function test and VDRL test

3. A 34-year-old primiparous woman is having generalized tonic–clonic convulsions. She is 32 weeks pregnant. Her blood pressure on arrival is 150/110 mmHg; she has 3+ proteinuria and she is still having convulsions. The fetal heart rate is reassuring. Which is the single most appropriate management? ★

A Diazepam and plan delivery

B Diazepam plus antihypertensive drug, and plan delivery

C Magnesium sulfate

D Magnesium sulfate plus antihypertensive drug

E Magnesium sulfate plus antihypertensive drug, and plan delivery

4. A 23-year-old woman is 34 weeks pregnant and has raised blood pressure. She is on 200 mg labetalol twice daily. Her blood pressure is 160/105 mmHg and she has 3+ proteinuria. She feels well, with no headaches or epigastric pain. The cardiotocograph (CTG) is reassuring. All blood tests are normal. Which is the single most appropriate management? ★

A Admit her to hospital for urgent delivery

B Admit her to hospital to stabilize her blood pressure

C Arrange for her to attend the day unit for twice-daily CTG

D Increase the labetalol dose, and follow up with the community midwife

E Increase the labetalol dose, and follow up in the day unit

5. A 32-year-old primipara is seen at 42 weeks' gestation. She is keen to go into labour naturally and refuses an induction of labour. Which is the single best reason to give for allowing induction of labour when counselling her? ★

A There is an increased risk of Caesarean section beyond 42 weeks' gestation

B There is an increased risk of intrauterine growth restriction beyond 42 weeks' gestation

C There is an increased risk of placental abruption beyond 42 weeks' gestation

D There is an increased risk of shoulder dystocia beyond 42 weeks' gestation

E There is an increased risk of unexplained fetal death beyond 42 weeks' gestation

6. The midwife on the delivery suite calls for help. A woman who has just had a normal delivery with active management of the third stage of labour is bleeding heavily. The bleeding started 15 minutes after delivery of the placenta. Her estimated blood loss is 900 mL. Her pulse rate is 95 bpm and her blood pressure is 100/55 mmHg. Which is the single most appropriate first-line management? ★

A Massage the uterus and give intramuscular (IM) carboprost (Haemabate®)

B Massage the uterus and give IM Syntocinon®

C Massage the uterus and start a Syntocinon® infusion

D Massage the uterus and start a blood transfusion

E Take the woman to theatre immediately for examination under anaesthesia

7. A 24-year-old woman has regular painful uterine contractions at 26 weeks' gestation. She is 2 cm dilated. Her membranes are intact. The cardiotocograph (CTG) is reassuring. Which is the single most appropriate management plan? ★

A Admit her, and administer analgesics and Syntocinon®

B Admit her, and administer antibiotics and intramuscular (IM) steroids

C Admit her, and administer antibiotics and tocolytic drugs

D Admit her, and administer tocolytic drugs and IM steroids

E Reassure her, and send her home

8. A para 4 is referred at 34 weeks of gestation to the antenatal day unit for parenteral iron therapy. Her haemoglobin is 6.9 mg/dL, with a ferritin of 3 micrograms/L. Her serum haemoglobin electrophoresis is normal. During administration of the parenteral iron, she develops headache, hypertension and wheeze. What is the single most important medication to give immediately after stopping the infusion? ★

A Adrenaline intramuscularly (IM) 1:1000 0.5 mL

B Chlorphenamine intravenously (IV) 10 mg

C Hydrocortisone IV 200 mg

D Paracetamol by mouth (PO) 1 g

E Salbutamol by nebulizer (NEB) 5 mL

9. A 26-year-old primigravida is in advanced labour. Her labour has been augmented using Syntocinon®, so a cardiotocograph (CTG) is performed. This is shown in Figure 1.1 (see Colour Plate section). Which is the single most appropriate management? ★ ★

A Perform urgent fetal blood sampling

B Perform an emergency Caesarean section

C Reassure the woman

D Stop the CTG recording

E Stop the Syntocinon® infusion

10. A 36-year-old woman who is human immunodeficiency virus (HIV)-positive discovers that she is pregnant. She is uncertain whether to continue the pregnancy, in particular because of the risk of the child acquiring her HIV infection. Her health is good and she has not yet needed to take antiretroviral therapy. If the pregnancy is managed appropriately, which is the single probability of her baby acquiring HIV infection? ★ ★

A 0% (i.e. no risk)

B Approximately 1%

C Approximately 15%

D Approximately 25%

E Approximately 40%

11. A 32-year-old primiparous woman is 'small for dates' at 34 weeks' gestation. An ultrasound scan shows a singleton fetus with an abdominal circumference at the 10th centile. The amniotic fluid volume and umbilical artery Dopplers are normal. Which is the single most appropriate management? ★ ★

A CTG monitoring on alternate days

B Reassure her that the baby is growing appropriately

C Repeat the ultrasound scan in 2 weeks' time

D Repeat the ultrasound scan in 4 weeks' time

E Urgent delivery by Caesarean section

12. A 42-year-old woman is 15 weeks pregnant and requests a quadruple test to rule out Down's syndrome. Which is the single most appropriate advice to give her? ★ ★

A It is too early in pregnancy to have the quadruple test

B It is too late in pregnancy to have the quadruple test

C She could have the quadruple test arranged today

D She must first agree to have an amniocentesis if the test is screen-positive

E The quadruple test will definitely be screen-positive because of her age

13. A 33-year-old woman has severe headache, blurred vision, abdominal pain and bleeding per vaginum at 33 weeks' gestation. The fetal heartbeat is absent. Which is the single most important associated clinical sign that may help in diagnosis? ★★

A Brisk tendon reflexes

B Enlarged thyroid gland

C Oedema

D Raised jugular venous pressure

E Tachycardia

14. A 29-year-old gravid 2 + 1 woman is 35 + 6 weeks pregnant. She has a history of a previous Caesarean section. She has had regular uterine contractions for 4 hours and a per vaginum 'show'. Following speculum examination, which is the single most appropriate management? ★★

A Cardiotocograph (CTG) monitoring

B Fibronectin test

C Intramuscular (IM) steroid

D Rescue cerclage

E Tocolysis

15. A primigravida presents to the delivery suite at 39 weeks' gestation with a history of regular contractions and rupture of membranes greater than 8 hours ago. On examination, she is 6 cm dilated. The cardiotocograph (CTG) is abnormal, therefore a fetal blood sample is collected. The pH is 7.018 and lactate 5.0 mmol/L. What is the single most appropriate management plan? ★★

A Deliver within 30 minutes

B Deliver within 60 minutes

C No action required

D Repeat sample after 30 minutes

E Repeat sample after 60 minutes

16. A 31-year-old para 1, with a history of a previous Caesarean section, is requesting a vaginal birth after Caesarean section (VBAC). She asks about the risk of problems. What single figure most accurately reflects the risk of scar dehiscence during labour? ★★★

A 0.5%

B 0.75%

C 1%

D 1.5%

E 2%

17. The midwife on the delivery suite calls for help. The fetal head has been delivered 2 minutes earlier and there is difficulty with delivery of the fetal shoulders. What is the single most effective manoeuvre to overcome this situation? ★★★

A Episiotomy

B Fundal pressure

C McRoberts' manoeuvre

D Suprapubic pressure

E Zavenelli manoeuvre

18. A 31-year-old primigravida, 29^{+3} weeks, presents to the antenatal clinic with reduced fetal movement for the last 6 hours. What is the single most appropriate initial investigation to confirm fetal viability? ★★★

A Biophysical profile

B Cardiotocography

C Doppler of umbilical artery

D Fetal movement chart

E Handheld Doppler

19. A 41-year-old primigravida presents to the antenatal clinic at 11^{+3} weeks' gestation, requesting a screening test for trisomy 21. Which is the single most sensitive and specific test available to her? ★★★

A Biophysical profile

B Cell free deoxyribonucleic acid (DNA) analysis

C Nuchal translucency test

D Triple test

E Quadruple test

20. A 27-year-old primigravida is seen at the antenatal clinic at term[+14]. The pregnancy has been uneventful and she is declining induction of labour. What is the single most appropriate management plan to ensure fetal well-being? ★ ★ ★

A Daily fetal kick chart monitoring

B Weekly biophysical profile

C Weekly amniotic fluid index and umbilical artery Doppler

D Twice-weekly cardiotocography (CTG) and amniotic fluid index

E Twice-weekly CTG and umbilical artery Doppler

21. A 19-year-old woman is taking carbamazepine as treatment for her epilepsy. She is 16 weeks pregnant. She had been fit-free for 5 years before becoming pregnant but has had two episodes of absence seizures in the past month. She has not informed the Driver and Vehicle Licensing Agency (DVLA) of her recent seizures. Which is the single most appropriate action to take at this stage? ★ ★ ★ ★

A Advise her to inform the DVLA immediately of her recent seizures

B Advise her to seek a second opinion about the safety of driving

C Inform the DVLA medical adviser immediately about the recent seizures

D Inform the patient's general practitioner (GP) about the recent seizures

E Reassure the patient that there is no need to inform the DVLA

22. A 22-year-old primigravida undergoes a Neville–Barnes forceps delivery. The fetal head is delivered in the occiput posterior (OP) position. On examination, the woman has a tear involving approximately one-third of the external anal sphincter thickness. What is the single most appropriate classification of this tear? ★ ★ ★ ★

A Second-degree tear

B Third-degree 3a tear

C Third-degree 3b tear

D Third-degree 3c tear

E Fourth-degree tear

23. A 21-year-old primigravida presents to the antenatal clinic with a breech presentation at 37^{+4} weeks' gestation. She is requesting an external cephalic version (ECV). What single drug treatment, given prior to ECV, is most effective at increasing the success rate? ★ ★ ★ ★

A Atosiban

B Glyceryl trinitrate

C Indomethacin

D Nifedipine

E Salbutamol

24. A 31-year-old primigravida presents to the labour ward at 31 weeks with a history of regular contractions. On vaginal examination, she is 2 cm dilated and the cervix is partially effaced. What is the single most cost-effective tocolytic treatment to give her? ★ ★ ★ ★

A Atosiban

B Indomethacin

C Magnesium sulfate

D Nifedipine

E Ritodrine

25. A 29-year-old, 31^{+4} weeks pregnant primigravida presents to the Emergency Department with a history of travel to rural India. On examination, her pulse is 118 bpm and blood pressure (BP) 90/60 mmHg, and her Glasgow Coma Scale (GCS) score is 11/15. She is diagnosed with falciparum malaria. What is the single most effective treatment option? ★ ★ ★ ★

A Artesunate

B Chloroquine

C Clindamycin

D Primaquine

E Quinine

26. A para 1^{+3} is reviewed in the high risk antenatal clinic at 32^{+2} weeks' gestation. She has an uncomplicated triplet pregnancy. What is the single most appropriate time to deliver this pregnancy? ★ ★ ★ ★

A 32 weeks' gestation

B 33 weeks' gestation

C 34 weeks' gestation

D 35 weeks' gestation

E 36 weeks' gestation

ANSWERS

1. B ★　　　OHCS 10th edn → p. 56

This woman is shocked. The abdominal pain and tense uterus suggest abruption. Blood loss may be concealed, so do not expect large amounts of visible bleeding. Placenta praevia is usually painless and the blood loss is greater, so it is often noticed earlier. There are no contractions, so labour has not started, although delivery will be expedited as the patient is unwell. A cervical ectropion may bleed but will not cause pain and shock.

2. B ★　　　OHCS 10th edn → p. 10

There are clear guidelines for antenatal care.
→ http://www.nice.org.uk/guidance/CG62

3. E ★　　　OHCS 10th edn → p. 49

Magnesium sulfate is the evidence-based treatment for eclamptic seizures. This patient also needs to have her blood pressure controlled carefully and delivery expedited.
→ http://www.nice.org.uk/guidance/cg107

4. B ★　　　OHCS 10th edn → p. 48

Although the patient is currently asymptomatic, her blood pressure is above 160/100 mmHg and she has significant proteinuria, despite labetalol treatment. She needs admission for careful monitoring and controlled management with antihypertensives, and consideration of delivery if there is no improvement.

5. E ★　　　OHCS 10th edn → pp. 54, 62

The reason why inductions are booked at 42 weeks is that the risk of intrauterine death increases significantly thereafter.

6. B ★　　　OHCS 10th edn → p. 84

Massaging the uterus helps to stimulate a contraction; the commonest cause is uterine atony. Syntocinon® IM is the first-line treatment. It is a synthetic version of oxytocin and stimulates contractions. If bleeding does not stop, Syntocinon® infusion and carboprost can be used, along with other approaches, for a major haemorrhage such as blood transfusion and fresh frozen plasma. Blood loss of over 1000 mL, or clinical signs of shock, are considered to represent a major incident.

7. D ★　　　OHCS 10th edn → p. 50

This woman has gone into premature labour, but this is at an early stage, so there is a possibility that it can be stopped with tocolytic drugs.

However, steroids should still be given to mature the fetal lungs in case delivery goes ahead. There is no indication of infection, so antibiotics are not routinely given.

→ http://www.nice.org.uk/guidance/ng25

8. A ★   OHCS 10th edn → p. 237

Patients having an anaphylactic reaction should be identified early and help sought immediately. The initial assessment and treatment should be based on the ABCDE (airway, breathing, circulation, disability, and exposure) approach. Pregnant women should be placed in the left lateral position to prevent aorto-caval compression. Stop any drug/trigger suspected of causing the reaction, then give adrenaline (epinephrine), administered as IM 1:1000 in a dose of 0.5 mL. The other medications will be needed after this, but adrenaline is lifesaving and should be given without delay.

→ http://www.resus.org.uk

9. C ★★   OHCS 10th edn → pp. 44–5

This is a normal CTG, with a baseline of 110–160 bpm, a variability of more than 5 bpm, and accelerations seen.

→ http://www.nice.org.uk/guidance/cg190/resources/interpretation-of-cardiotocograph-traces-248732173

10. B ★★   OHCS 10th edn → p. 22

The risks associated with modern management using antiretroviral drugs and elective Caesarean section are very low, although they are not eliminated completely.

11. C ★★   OHCS 10th edn → p. 52

Serial ultrasound scans to detect changes in abdominal circumference are accurate in diagnosing growth restriction. As this baby's abdominal circumference is less than the 10th centile, it may be growth-restricted, and a scan should be repeated after 2 weeks.

→ http://www.rcog.org.uk/en/guidelines-research-services/guidelines/gtg31/

12. C ★★   OHCS 10th edn → p. 14

The quadruple test measures maternal serum levels of α-fetoprotein, human chorionic gonadotrophin and unconjugated oestriol, interpreted along with a dating scan. It uses these values, together with maternal age, to calculate the risk of certain conditions. It is a screening tool and is not diagnostic. If the risk is high, the mother can, if she wishes, choose further diagnostic tests.

13. A ★★   OHCS 10th edn → p. 48

These symptoms indicate severe pre-eclampsia. Brisk reflexes are commonly associated with pre-eclampsia. The others are just general clinical signs.

14. A ★★   OHCS 10th edn → p. 60

This woman may be in labour, and the single most appropriate plan of management in her case will involve a speculum examination and CTG to assess this. It is inappropriate to insert a cerclage at this gestation. A fibronectin test is contraindicated if there is bleeding per vaginum. A single course of antenatal corticosteroids is administered to women between 24^{+0} and 34^{+6} weeks' gestation.

→ http://www.nice.org.uk/guidance/ng25

15. A ★★   OHCS 10th edn → p. 46

Fetal blood sampling is done to give a sign of how distressed a fetus is. An acidotic sample with a high lactate indicates a high level of distress and should be acted upon. The recommended intervention cut-off value for lactate is 4.8 mmol/L.

Above this, the fetus should be delivered immediately, by either instrument or urgent Caesarean section.

→ http://www.nice.org.uk/guidance/cg190/resources/intrapartum-care-for-healthy-women-and-babies-35109866447557

16. A ★★★   OHCS 10th edn → p. 80

Women should be informed that a planned VBAC is associated with an approximately 1:200 (0.5%) risk of uterine rupture. The success rate for a vaginal delivery after a previous Caesarean section (VBAC) is 72–75%.

→ http://www.rcog.org.uk/globalassets/documents/guidelines/gtg_45.pdf

17. C ★★★   OHCS 10th edn → p. 72

An episiotomy is not always necessary, and maternal pushing should be discouraged as this may impact fetal shoulders further. Fundal pressure should not be used and is associated with high fetal and maternal complication rates, including uterine rupture. The McRoberts' manoeuvre consists of flexion and abduction of the mother's hips, placing her thighs onto her abdomen. The reported success rates for this manoeuvre is 90% and therefore should be employed first. If this fails to correct the problem, other manoeuvres can be used: applying pressure to the posterior aspect of the anterior shoulder (suprapubic pressure) or internal manipulations. In the Zavenelli manoeuvre, the fetal head is replaced into the birth canal and the fetus is rescued abdominally, but this has a high mortality rate so is a last resort.

→ http:///www.rcog.org.uk/globalassets/documents/guidelines/gtg_42.pdf

18. E ★ ★ ★   OHCS 10th edn → p. 4

A handheld Doppler will, in most cases, confirm the presence of a fetal heartbeat. This is widely available in most settings. If the fetal heartbeat is not confirmed, then immediate referral for an ultrasound scan to assess fetal cardiac activity is required.

After viability has been confirmed, if the woman still complains of reduced fetal movement, then a CTG should be performed. If she continues to complain of reduced fetal movements, and despite having a normal CTG, then a detailed ultrasound scan should be undertaken.

→ http://www.rcog.org.uk/globalassets/documents/guidelines/gtg_57.pdf

19. B ★ ★ ★   OHCS 10th edn → p. 15

Cell free DNA analysis works by analysing, counting and mapping the DNA fragments that are present in maternal plasma during pregnancy and can be performed from about 10 weeks. It has a less than 0.1% false positive rate for trisomies 21, 18 and 13. Fewer than 1 in 1000 non-invasive prenatal testing (NIPT) tests yield a false positive result. The detection rate for conventional screening tests, including quadruple screen, is 81%. A first-trimester screen with a nuchal transluceny scan is 85%. Integrated screening gives a 95% detection rate. The biophysical profile is not a screening test.

→ Juneau K, Bogard PE, Huang S, et al. Microarray-based cell-free DNA analysis improves noninvasive prenatal testing. *Fetal Diagn Ther.* 2014;**36**:282–6.

20. D ★ ★ ★   OHCS 10th edn → p. 62

Women with uncomplicated pregnancies should be offered induction of labour at 41 weeks. After 42 weeks, if a woman declines induction, then the health of the fetus should be monitored. She should be offered at least twice-weekly CTG and ultrasound estimation of the maximum amniotic pool depth. These best monitor fetal distress and placental function.

→ http://www.nice.org.uk/guidance/cg62/resources/antenatal-care-for-uncomplicated-pregnancies-975564597445

21. A ★ ★ ★ ★

Patients who have had a seizure should refrain from driving for 1 year. It is the patient's responsibility to inform the DVLA, which may then seek information from the doctor. However, the doctor should inform the patient of this requirement, as they may be unaware of it.

→ http://www.epilepsysociety.org.uk/driving-regulations

22. B ★ ★ ★ ★   OHCS 10th edn → p. 92

It is important to recognize and appropriately treat perineal tears in order to prevent future morbidity, particularly anal incontinence. Risk factors for tears include primiparity, large babies (>4 kg), occiput posterior (OP)

position, induction, epidural use, prolonged second stage, forceps use and midline episiotomy.

Classification is as follows:*

- first degree: injury to the perineal skin only
- second degree: injury to the perineum involving the perineal muscles, but not the anal sphincter
- third degree: injury to the perineum involving the anal sphincter complex, consisting of the external anal sphincter (EAS) and internal anal sphincter (IAS):
  - 3a: less than 50% of EAS thickness torn
  - 3b: more than 50% of EAS thickness torn
  - 3c: both EAS and IAS torn
- fourth degree: injury to the perineum involving the anal sphincter complex (EAS and IAS) and anal epithelium.

→ http://www.rcog.org.uk/en/guidelines-research-services/guidelines/gtg29/

23. E ★★★★   OHCS 10th edn → p. 70

Women should be counselled that, with a trained operator, about 50% of ECV attempts will be successful. ECV success rates are increased by the use of tocolysis. The drugs shown to be effective include ritodrine, salbutamol and terbutaline.

→ http://www.rcog.org.uk/globalassets/documents/guidelines/gt20aexternalcephalicversion.pdf

24. D ★★★★   OHCS 10th edn → p. 50

Nifedipine and atosiban have comparable effectiveness in delaying birth up to 7 days. Ritodrine and atosiban are licensed in the United Kingdom (UK) for treatment of pre-term labour. Although the use of nifedipine for pre-term labour is an unlicensed indication, it is associated with improved neonatal outcomes and is therefore in use. It is also orally administered, and the cost for a standard 48-hour treatment with nifedipine is £1, as compared with £494 for atosiban.

→ https://www.nice.org.uk/guidance/ng25

25. A ★★★★   OHCS 10th edn → p. 26

Admit women with complicated malaria and treat it as an emergency. Intravenous artesunate is the treatment of choice for severe falciparum malaria, including in pregnant women. Intravenous quinine can be used if artesunate is not available. Primaquine should not be used in pregnancy.

*Adapted from: Royal College of Obstetricians and Gynaecologists. *The Management of Third- and Fourth-Degree Perineal Tears.* Green-top Guideline No. 29. London: RCOG; 2015, with the permission of the Royal College of Obstetricians and Gynaecologists.

Quinine and clindamycin can be used to treat uncomplicated *Plasmodium falciparum* or *Plasmodium vivax*.

→ http://www.rcog.org.uk/globalassets/documents/guidelines/gtg_54b.pdf

26. B ★★★★ OHCS 10th edn → p. 68

Triplet pregnancies should be offered elective delivery by Caesarean section from 35 weeks' gestation, after a course of antenatal corticosteroids. Seventy-five per cent of triplet pregnancies will result in spontaneous labour before 35 weeks 0 days. Delivery too early puts the infants at more risk of complications so should be avoided.

→ http://www.nice.org.uk/guidance/cg129/resources/multiple-pregnancy-antenatal-care-for-twin-and-triplet-pregnancies-35109458300869

Paediatrics

Luci Etheridge

Children are not merely small adults. To be a good paediatrician requires as much knowledge about health as about disease. The normal patterns of growth and development can be a mystery to many, and paediatricians are often called upon to help to interpret these for confused parents. There is a unique need to be aware of the range of congenital disorders that may present before, at, or shortly after birth. Younger children cannot tell us their symptoms. Therefore, paediatricians have to learn to pick up on non-verbal clues and often subtle signs, when the answer may lie in something unexpected and far removed from the traditional history and examination format. At the other end of the spectrum, adolescents have their own range of health issues and are traditionally an under-represented and often forgotten group. In this chapter, we aim to cover many of the key presentations and issues in children of all ages, from neonates to teenagers.

Even in this modern age, children are susceptible to infection. Respiratory and gastrointestinal infections are the commonest presentations in both general practice and paediatric hospital practice. Fortunately, most of these infections are self-limiting, but serious infections do occur and must be recognized. However, the leading cause of death in all children over 1 year of age is accidents. Recognizing risk factors for accidental and non-accidental harm is a major responsibility for all those working with children.

The questions in this chapter will test not only the common areas that present to paediatricians, but also relevant issues such as knowledge of disease factors, ethics, and risk management in relation to children and their families. However, the best way to learn about children is to get out there and meet them—play with them, talk to their parents and carers, and see them when they are ill and well. You will learn the most this way and be able to apply that knowledge and experience to answer questions such as these.

QUESTIONS

1. A 1-day-old girl has a harsh systolic cardiac murmur all over the precordium, with a thrill at the left sternal edge. Femoral pulses are palpable. A chest X-ray shows an enlarged heart, and an electrocardiogram (ECG) shows left ventricular hypertrophy. Which is the single most likely diagnosis? ★

A Aortic stenosis

B Coarctation of the aorta

C Patent ductus arteriosus

D Pulmonary stenosis

E Ventricular septal defect

2. A 4-month-old boy is due to have his routine immunization. After the last set of immunizations, he had a 2-cm red area on his thigh around the injection site and seemed irritable for several hours. He has had a runny nose for the last 2 days, but no fever. His mother asks whether it is all right to proceed with his immunizations. Which is the single most appropriate piece of advice to give? ★

A Postpone immunization until his runny nose has settled

B Immunize him in hospital

C Omit pertussis, but proceed with the other immunizations

D Omit this set of immunizations

E Reassure the mother and proceed with the planned immunizations now

3. A 7-year-old girl is drowsy and panting, and has a capillary blood glucose level of 25 mmol/L and ketones and protein in her urine. Initial blood results show:

- sodium 145 mmol/L
- potassium 3.8 mmol/L
- creatinine 100 µmol/L
- urea 12 mmol/L
- calcium 2.6 mmol/L
- glucose 26 mmol/L.

She is given two fluid boluses of 10 mL/kg 0.9% saline and is then started on a 0.9% saline infusion to deliver a total of maintenance plus 10% over 48 hours. Intravenous (IV) insulin is also started. Two hours later, she has improved, has passed urine, and is more alert. Her blood results show:

- sodium 143 mmol/L
- potassium 3.8 mmol/L
- creatinine 82 µmol/L
- urea 10 mmol/L
- calcium 2.2 mmol/L
- glucose 20 mmol/L.

Which single fluid should she now be given IV? ★

A 0.45% saline and 5% dextrose

B 0.45% saline and 5% dextrose with added calcium

C 0.45% saline and 5% dextrose with added potassium

D 0.9% saline

E 0.9% saline with added potassium

4. A 5-year-old girl had been passing hard stools once every 5 to 7 days for 6 months. She was started on two Movicol® Paediatric sachets daily. She continued this treatment for 1 month and started passing a stool every day, so her parents stopped it. For the last month, she has been soiling her pants, with intermittent runny stools. She opens her bowels on the toilet most days and passes pellet-like stools and an occasional large, hard stool. Which is the single main deficiency in her management so far? ★

A Colonoscopy should have been performed

B Glycerol suppositories should have been added

C Movicol® should have been continued for several more months

D She should have had an enema when she was first seen

E Stimulant laxatives should have been used

5. A 7-year-old boy wets the bed most nights and has never been reliably dry. He is a heavy sleeper. He has kept a star chart for 4 weeks and his parents have been supportive. His chart shows one dry night each week, with no particular pattern. He has a cub camp in 4 months' time. Urinalysis is negative. Which is the single most appropriate management? ★

A Star chart

B Enuresis alarm

C Desmopressin melts at night

D Imipramine tablets at night

E Oxybutynin tablets at night

6. A 1-year-old boy has had diarrhoea for the past 12 hours. At the beginning of the illness, he vomited twice. He has not passed urine for the past 6 hours. He is thirsty and restless, his eyes are sunken, the mucous membranes are dry, and skin turgor has decreased. His pulse rate is 160 bpm, and his capillary refill time is 2 seconds. Which is the single best description of his degree of dehydration and the appropriate initial fluid to give? ★

A Mild; oral rehydration solution

B Mild; 0.9% saline intravenously (IV)

C Moderate; oral rehydration solution

D Moderate; 0.9% saline IV

E Severe; 0.9% saline IV

7. A 20-hour-old term newborn boy has a short soft early systolic murmur on his baby check. He is pink, with no signs of respiratory distress, and has normally palpable femoral pulses and a normal apex beat. The murmur is heard at the upper left sternal edge and radiates through the chest. There are no associated heaves or thrills. Which is the single most likely diagnosis? ★

A Atrial septal defect

B Innocent heart murmur

C Patent ductus arteriosus

D Pulmonary stenosis

E Ventricular septal defect

8. A 12-year-old girl, who recently arrived in the United Kingdom from South Asia, has had pain and swelling of both knees, ankles, and wrists for 5 days, and these symptoms come and go. Five weeks ago, she had a cold and a sore throat. For the last day, she has had a rash on her trunk, which has a pink border and is fading centrally. Both knees have an effusion and limited flexion to 70°. The girl's temperature is 39.2°C and her pulse rate is 160 bpm. Which single organism is likely to be responsible for this illness? ★

A *Corynebacterium diphtheriae*

B Human cytomegalovirus

C Epstein–Barr virus

D Group A β-haemolytic *Streptococcus*

E *Staphylococcus aureus*

9. A 6-year-old boy has had vomiting for 24 hours and has been unable to keep any liquids down, although he has not wanted to eat any food. Today he has central abdominal pain, which was coming and going but is now constant and sharp. He has pain when he tries to pass urine and gets very upset if he is moved. He has opened his bowels once today and passed a loose stool. Which is the single most likely diagnosis? ★

A Appendicitis

B Gastro-oesophageal reflux

C Mesenteric adenitis

D Viral gastroenteritis

E Volvulus

10. A 39-week-gestation baby girl, who weighs 3.4 kg, is due for her baby check. She is lying supine. The examiner's left hand is stabilizing the pelvis and his right hand is grasping the left leg, flexed at the hip and knee, with his thumb over the lesser trochanter and the tip of his middle finger over the greater trochanter. He wants first to check whether the right hip is dislocatable with Barlow's manoeuvre. Which is the single most accurate description of how the examination should be performed? ★

A Adduct the leg to the midline and apply gentle anterior pressure over the greater trochanter

B Adduct the leg to the midline and apply gentle posterior pressure over the lesser trochanter

C Fully abduct the leg and apply gentle posterior pressure over the lesser trochanter

D Fully abduct the leg and apply gentle anterior pressure over the greater trochanter

E Partially abduct the leg and apply gentle anterior pressure over the greater trochanter

11. A 24-month-old girl enjoys 'feeding' her dolls. She does not like taking turns. She is able to walk upstairs with help but is unable to stand on one leg. She is able to scribble but is unable to draw a circle. She can say 'mama' and 'dada' with meaning, but no other recognizable words. In which single developmental area is she showing delay? ★

A Fine motor skills

B Gross motor skills

C Social skills

D Speech and language skills

E Play skills

12. A 14-year-old girl has chronic kidney disease. Her nephrologist advises that dialysis is the only option while she is awaiting renal transplant. She refuses to have dialysis and appears to understand the consequence of not having treatment. She was in and out of local authority care between the ages of 1 and 6 years but has been living with her parents for the last 8 years. Her mother, who has sole parental responsibility, wants her to have dialysis, but her father feels that she should decide for herself. The family have been through extensive counselling with the team but have not been able to reach a consensus. Which single decision takes precedence when deciding further management? ★

A That of the father

B That of the local authority

C That of the mother

D That of the nephrologist

E That of the patient

13. A 2-month-old boy has faltering growth. He is a sweaty baby, particularly during breastfeeding. He has a palpable 4-cm liver edge. He is pale and has a respiratory rate of 60 breaths/minute, a heart rate of 180 bpm, and a blood pressure of 80/40 mmHg, and his oxygen saturation is 96% in air. His capillary refill time is 3 seconds, and his capillary blood glucose concentration is 5 mmol/L. Which single system of the body is most likely to be affected? ★

A Cardiovascular system

B Gastrointestinal system

C Metabolic system

D Neurological system

E Respiratory system

14. A 37-week-gestation baby who weighed 2.7 kg at birth is now 4 days old. He is being breastfed. During the first 24 hours of life, he did not latch on to the breast well and fed for approximately 5 minutes at a time every 4 to 5 hours. He is now feeding for 15–20 minutes every 2 to 3 hours. His weight today is 2.55 kg. His mother is worried about his weight loss. Which is the single most appropriate advice to give her? ★

A Any weight loss in the first week is worrying, and he should have supplementary feeds

B He has lost less than 10% of his birthweight, which is acceptable in the first week, and she should continue breastfeeding

C He has lost less than 10% of his birthweight, which is acceptable in the first week, but he should have supplementary feeds until he gains weight

D He has lost more than 10% of his birthweight, which is acceptable in the first week, and she should continue breastfeeding

E He has lost more than 10% of his birthweight, which is more than is normal in the first week, so he should have supplementary feeds

15. A 14-year-old Caucasian boy has had raised temperatures with drenching night sweats and malaise for 8 weeks. He has lost 4 kg in weight. He had a ventricular septal defect repaired in infancy. He looks pale, has extensive dental decay, and has small, linear areas of bleeding under his nail beds. He has a three-finger-breadth splenomegaly and a grade 2 systolic murmur, heard best on the lower left sternal edge. His temperature is 38°C. Which is the single most appropriate treatment? ★

A Antibiotics

B Chemotherapy

C Diuretics

D High-dose steroids

E Surgery

16. An 18-month-old African-Caribbean girl is not yet walking. She was breastfed for 9 months and is thriving along the 25th centile for weight. She has bow legs, Harrison's sulci, and swollen wrists. Which single vitamin deficiency is she most likely to have? ★

A Vitamin A

B Vitamin B_{12}

C Vitamin C

D Vitamin D

E Vitamin E

17. A mother brings her 7-month-old boy to the Emergency Department. She says he is always 'on the go', and that morning he fell out of his cot onto the laminate flooring, from a height of approximately 3 feet. He is now not moving his right leg. He has a spiral fracture of the right femur on X-ray. Which single part of the history will help most in deciding further management? ★

A Birth history

B Family medical history

C Developmental history

D Social history

E Systems review questioning

18. A 4-year-old Caucasian boy has poorly controlled asthma, despite being on a high-dose steroid inhaler and a leukotriene receptor antagonist and compliant with his medication. He has recurrent chest infections and has significant nasal discharge. He also has poor growth, Harrison's sulci, and finger clubbing. Which is the single most appropriate next investigation? ★

A Bronchial brush biopsy

B Bronchoalveolar lavage

C Computed tomography (CT) scan of the chest

D Lung function tests

E Sweat test

19. A 4-year-old boy has periorbital oedema, central abdominal discomfort, and decreased urine output. His urine dipstick shows 3+ proteinuria and no blood. He is asthmatic and recently had a bad 'cold.' Which is the single most likely diagnosis? ★

A Angio-oedema

B Nephrotic syndrome

C Post-streptococcal glomerulonephritis

D Postural proteinuria

E Systemic lupus erythematosus (SLE)

20. A 7-year-old boy with asthma has had a 'cold' and a temperature of 37.7°C for 24 hours. He has severe respiratory distress and requires 15 L/minute of oxygen to maintain his oxygen saturation above 95%. He is started on nebulized salbutamol therapy, which causes an initial improvement in his symptoms. He then suddenly deteriorates, with marked respiratory distress, hypoxia, and hypotension. Which is the single most likely diagnosis? ★

A Anaphylaxis

B Pleural effusion

C Pneumonia

D Pulmonary embolus

E Tension pneumothorax

21. A 6-year-old girl has had vomiting and central abdominal pain for 3 days. She has eczema and poorly controlled asthma. She looks pale and has a Glasgow Coma Scale score of 11/15. Her abdomen is generally tender, but there is no rigidity, rebound, or guarding. Bowel sounds are present and normal. Her respiratory rate is 36 breaths/minute, with no recession. Her heart rate is 160 bpm and her capillary refill time is 4 seconds. She is given a 20 mL/kg bolus of fluid. Blood tests show:

- haemoglobin 13 g/dL
- white cell count 22×10^9/L
- C-reactive protein 25 mg/L
- sodium 120 mmol/L
- potassium 6.8 mmol/L
- urea 9.3 mmol/L
- creatinine 110 μmol/L.

Which is the single most important next investigation? ★

A Abdominal ultrasound scan

B Blood glucose

C Computed tomography (CT) scan of the head

D Serum ammonia

E Urine osmolality

22. A 3-year-old boy is in acute respiratory distress. There is no past history of note, except that he has not been immunized. He has a temperature of 40°C, looks flushed and unwell, is drooling, and has an inspiratory stridor. His cough is muffled. A colleague asks for help examining the boy's throat. Which is the single most appropriate advice to give? ★

A Do not disturb the child, and call for senior help urgently

B Give nebulized budesonide, and then examine the throat

C Go ahead and examine the throat, but have a laryngoscope and an endotracheal tube to hand

D Go ahead and examine the throat straight away to help to make a diagnosis

E Site an intravenous line and give a dose of cefotaxime first, and then examine the throat

23. A 9-month-old boy has had a generalized seizure, which lasted for 5 minutes, during which he stared straight ahead and his arms and legs shook. He had been unwell for 12 hours with fever, a runny nose, and cough. He has never had any fits before, and there is no family history of epilepsy. His development had been appropriate for his age, but in the last 6 weeks he has stopped pulling to stand or cruising round furniture. His temperature is 39°C and he has pharyngitis. A diagnosis of febrile convulsion is made. Which single feature in the history is least consistent with a diagnosis of febrile convulsion? ★

A The absence of previous febrile fits

B The age of the child

C The description of the seizure

D The developmental history

E The duration of the seizure

24. A 3-month-old baby girl has dry skin on her scalp, as shown in Figure 2.1 (see Colour Plate section). It has been present for the past 5 weeks and is getting progressively worse. Which is the single most likely diagnosis? ★

A Atopic eczema

B Impetigo

C Psoriasis

D Seborrhoeic dermatitis

E Tinea capitis

25. A 2.8-kg, 37-week-gestation baby girl has been treated briefly with phototherapy for jaundice. She is now 7 days old, breast-feeding well, and starting to regain weight. She has been off photo-therapy for over 48 hours, and her bilirubin chart is shown in Figure 2.2 (see Colour Plate section). Her mother has heard someone mention that her baby has 'breast milk jaundice' and wants to know how she should continue to feed her baby. Which is the single most appropriate advice to give the mother? ★★

A She should continue to breastfeed, but also give some extra formula feeds to ensure a good milk intake to help to reduce the jaundice

B She should continue to breastfeed exclusively, as this is still the best milk for her baby, regardless of the jaundice, which is already improving

C She should give mainly formula milk for the next 3 weeks, with the occasional breastfeed to ensure an ongoing breast milk supply

D She should stop breastfeeding completely and change to a term for-mula to prevent the jaundice from worsening again

E She should stop breastfeeding for 48 hours to allow the jaundice level to fall further, and then restart

26. A 20-month-old South Asian boy has bow legs. He was breastfed until the age of 6 months. The family live in a sixth-floor, two-bedroom flat, and his mother wears the hijab. He has mild genu varum bilaterally. His wrist X-ray is shown in Figure 2.3 (see Colour Plate section). Which single area of the X-ray shows the bony abnormal-ities that indicate the likely diagnosis? ★★

A Carpal bones

B Diaphyses of long bones

C Epiphyses of long bones

D Metacarpal bones

E Metaphyses of long bones

27. A 7-year-old girl has had general malaise and pallor for the past 3 days. She is passing small amounts of urine infrequently. She was unwell the previous week with bloody diarrhoea, but this has now settled. Blood results show:

- haemoglobin 8.2 g/dL
- platelets 400 × 10⁹/L
- white cell count 10.4 × 10⁹/L
- sodium 135 mmol/L
- potassium 4.2 mmol/L
- urea 22 mmo/L
- creatinine 230 μmol/L
- C-reactive protein 11 mg/L.

Which single organism is the most likely cause of her illness? ★ ★

A *Clostridium difficile*

B *Escherichia coli*

C *Salmonella typhi*

D *Shigella sonnei*

E *Streptococcus pneumoniae*

28. An 8-year-old boy has had headaches for 12 months. They are usually left-sided and throbbing and are made worse by noise and light. They last for around 12 hours, during which time he is nauseated but does not vomit. There are no obvious triggers. Treatment with paracetamol during attacks is of some benefit. He has one bad attack every 3 weeks on average, missing 1 to 2 days of school each time. Which is the single most appropriate next step in management? ★ ★

A Anti-emetic during attacks

B Computed tomography (CT) scan of the head

C Oral propranolol

D Psychology referral

E Sumatriptan nasal spray

29. A 15-year-old boy is worried that he is shorter than all his friends and that he has not yet started puberty. He is otherwise well. His father started puberty at around the age of 14 years. The boy's parental heights are both on the 25th centile. His growth chart is shown in Figure 2.4 (see Colour Plate section). Which single aspect of his growth and pubertal development will be most likely to assist with diagnosis? ★ ★

A Axillary hair stage

B Height centile

C Height velocity centile

D Pubic hair stage

E Testicular size

30. A 5-year-old boy returned from visiting relatives in Bangladesh a week ago. He has had a temperature of 39°C, lower abdominal pain, and loose stool for 5 days. Blood tests show:

- haemoglobin 10.6 g/dL
- white cell count 17×10^9/L
- lymphocyte count 13×10^9/L
- platelet count 400×10^9/L
- Gram-negative bacilli on blood culture.

Which is the single most likely diagnosis? ★ ★

A Dengue fever

B Leishmaniasis

C Leptospirosis

D Malaria

E Typhoid

31. A 4-month-old baby girl has had a temperature of 38°C for 2 days and is consuming less than half of her usual amount during feeding. She has had an irritable cry and has been very unsettled for the last 24 hours. She has had three loose stools and two vomiting episodes in the last 12 hours. A lumbar puncture is performed which shows:

- clear colourless cerebrospinal fluid (CSF)
- glucose 2.9 mmol/L (blood glucose 5.4 mmol/L)
- protein 32 mg/dL
- white cell count 60/mm³ (90% mononuclear cells)
- red cell count 10/mm³
- Gram-negative staining.

In travenous (IV) access is established and she is started on IV ceftriaxone. Which is the single most appropriate medication to add? ★ ★

A IV aciclovir

B IV metronidazole

C Oral dexamethasone

D Oral isoniazid

E Oral rifampicin

32. A 25-week-gestation infant has just been delivered by spontaneous vaginal delivery. The full neonatal resuscitation team is present and the Resuscitaire® has been pre-warmed. The baby is handed to the team and they have started the clock. Which is the single most important action to take next? ★ ★ ★

A Assess the baby's initial Apgar score

B Dry the baby thoroughly and check the heart rate

C Intubate immediately and start ventilation breaths

D Put a hat on the baby's head and a plastic bag over his body

E Suction the mouth under direct vision using a laryngoscope

33. A 14-year-old girl has an osteosarcoma of her tibia. She has worsening pain in her leg. She is on regular oral paracetamol and ibuprofen. Which is the single most appropriate next treatment? ★ ★ ★

A Codeine phosphate

B Diazepam

C Diclofenac

D Hyoscine bromide

E Morphine sulfate

34. A newborn baby boy has a urethral meatus that emerges on the dorsum of the penis, as shown in Figure 2.5 (see Colour Plate section). He is able to pass a good stream of urine. Which single piece of advice should be given to his parents before discharge? ★ ★ ★

A He should not be circumcised

B He should not wear disposable nappies

C The foreskin should be retracted gently every day

D The penis should be cleaned with mild soapy water daily

E This is entirely normal and no further measures are needed

35. A 4-year-old boy was accidentally given intravenous (IV) cefuroxime 30 minutes ago, which was prescribed on the wrong drug chart. He has no relevant allergies and does not seem to have suffered any ill effects. The antibiotic has been crossed off his chart. His parents have now returned to the ward after being at home. Which is the single most appropriate course of action? ★ ★ ★

A Discuss the error at handover later in the day and write a reflective portfolio entry

B Do nothing further until the error has been discussed with a medical defence organization

C Explain the error and apologize to the parents and notify a senior colleague promptly

D Notify a senior colleague with a view to explaining the error to the parents later in the day

E Shred the incorrect prescription chart and write a new one

36. A 4-month-old girl has been irritable, with a temperature of 38°C for 2 days. She is diagnosed with a coliform urinary tract infection (UTI). Blood and cerebrospinal fluid cultures are negative. She responds to oral antibiotics and is afebrile after 24 hours. Which single set of investigations should be performed (Table 2.1)? ★ ★ ★

Table 2.1 Investigation options

	Ultrasound of kidneys, ureters, and bladder	Dimercaptosuccinic acid (DMSA) renal isotope scan	Micturating cystourethrogram
A	No	No	No
B	Yes	No	No
C	Yes	Yes	No
D	Yes	No	Yes
E	Yes	Yes	Yes

37. A 14-year-old South Asian girl has had polyuria and polydipsia for 4 months. She has a body mass index of 28 kg/m² and dark, velvety pigmentation of the skin in her axillae. She has a random serum glucose concentration of 12 mmol/L and no blood ketones. Which is the single most likely diagnosis? ★ ★ ★

A Cushing's syndrome

B Diabetes insipidus

C Simple obesity

D Type 1 diabetes mellitus

E Type 2 diabetes mellitus

38. A 30-week-gestation infant is now 12 hours old. She was in good condition at birth and did not require resuscitation, although she did have some mild subcostal recession and needed 25% incubator oxygen. Over the past few hours, she has developed increasing respiratory distress, with grunting, intercostal and subcostal recession, and an increasing oxygen requirement to 45%. Her blood gas analysis shows a respiratory acidosis, and her chest X-ray has a homogeneous ground-glass appearance with air bronchograms. She has just been in-tubated. Which is the single most appropriate medication to give immediately? ★ ★ ★

A Amoxicillin intravenously (IV)

B Dexamethasone IV

C Gentamicin IV

D Morphine infusion IV

E Surfactant via an endotracheal tube

39. A 6-year-old boy is 'always on the go' and finds it difficult to take turns. He is easily distracted and finds it difficult to focus on any task. His father says that he has no sense of danger and often runs across the main road without any care. He has difficulty following a series of simple instructions and is 1 year behind his peers in his numeracy and literacy skills. Which is the single most likely diagnosis? ★ ★ ★

A Attention-deficit/hyperactivity disorder (ADHD)

B Autism

C Dyspraxia

D Global developmental delay

E Oppositional defiant disorder

40. A 38-week-gestation, 3.1-kg baby is delivered by spontaneous vaginal delivery. The pregnancy has been complicated by polyhydramnios. At birth, there are copious oral secretions and respiratory distress. The baby requires intubation and ventilation for respiratory distress and continues to drool. It is not possible to pass a nasogastric tube to the estimated length required, and no acid reaction is obtained. Chest X-ray shows the nasogastric tube coiled in the oesophagus, a moderately large stomach bubble, and a normal gas pattern in the bowel. Which is the single most likely diagnosis? ★ ★ ★ ★

A H-type tracheo-oesophageal fistula

B Isolated oesophageal atresia

C Oesophageal atresia and tracheo-oesophageal fistula

D Oesophageal stenosis

E Oesophageal stricture

41. An 8-year-old boy had a throat infection and was given penicillin 2 days ago. He now has a red rash, which is peeling, on his trunk and sore red eyes, and has developed lesions on his mouth, shown in Figure 2.6 (see Colour Plate section). He looks unwell and has a temperature of 39°C and a heart rate of 175 bpm. Which is the single most likely diagnosis? ★ ★ ★ ★

A Bullous impetigo

B Chickenpox

C Hand, foot, and mouth disease

D Measles

E Stevens–Johnson syndrome

42. A 9-week-old girl has had brief seizures for the last day, during which she stares straight ahead, her body shakes for a few seconds, and her right hand twitches. Pregnancy was normal, but delivery was difficult due to shoulder dystocia. Her Apgar scores were 7 at 1 minute and 9 at 5 minutes. She has some pale areas of skin over her right thigh. She is afebrile. Urea and electrolytes, calcium, magnesium, and glucose are all normal. Lumbar puncture is bloodstained, with a protein concentration of 0.97 g/L (normal range is up to 0.4 g/L). Her electroencephalogram (EEG) is normal. Her magnetic resonance imaging (MRI) brain scan is shown in Figure 2.7 (see Colour Plate section). Which is the single most likely diagnosis? ★★★★

A Benign neonatal seizures

B Hypoxic–ischaemic birth injury

C Infantile spasms

D Subdural haematoma

E Tuberous sclerosis

43. Five boys attend the same nursery. They are all aged 2 years 0 months and, by chance, they all have the same weight of 12.5 kg (50th centile). Their parents compare their birthweights and gestations, which are listed in Table 2.2. Which single child is most at risk of later obesity? ★★★★

Table 2.2 Birthweights and gestations

	Birthweight (centile)	Gestation (weeks)
A	1.5 kg (<0.4th)	40
B	1.5 kg (50th)	30
C	2.0 kg (98th)	30
D	3.5 kg (50th)	40
E	5.0 kg (99.6th)	40

44. A 48-hour-old, 2.8-kg term baby girl has pallor, poor perfusion, cyanosis, and respiratory distress. She was born in good condition and was well for the first few hours of life. She has been intubated and ventilated, but her oxygen saturations remain in the range of 70–80%, despite 100% oxygen and good chest movement. Her femoral pulses are not palpable. Which is the single most appropriate medication to commence next? ★ ★ ★ ★

A Dobutamine

B Dopamine

C Indomethacin

D Prostaglandin E$_2$

E Surfactant

45. A 4-year-old boy has had generalized oedema for 2 days and has 3+ proteinuria on dipstick testing of his urine. His blood pressure is 73/36 mmHg. His plasma albumin level is 18 g/L. All other blood tests, including his urea and electrolytes, are normal. He is started on high-dose daily oral prednisolone. Which single likelihood is there that he will respond to the treatment and not have any further relapses? ★ ★ ★ ★

A 3%

B 30%

C 50%

D 70%

E 90%

ANSWERS

1. E ★ OHCS 10th edn → p. 137

Heart murmurs are heard in many neonates. It is important to know the characteristics that signify congenital heart disease. Significant murmurs are usually harsh-sounding and may be associated with thrills. In this case, the systolic murmur indicates a lesion where turbulent flow occurs in systole (i.e. aortic stenosis, pulmonary stenosis, ventricular septal defect, and atrial septal defect). The thrill at the left sternal edge indicates turbulent flow in the area of the septum. A patent ductus has a continuous murmur as blood flows across the ductus in both systole and diastole. Normal femoral pulses argue against a severe aortic stenosis or coarctation.

For an excellent learning resource on congenital heart disease that explains the anatomy by likening it to the rooms of a house, see the Children's Heart Institute website:

→ http://childrensheartinstitute.org/educate/eduhome.htm

2. E ★ OHCS 10th edn → p. 151

The mild upper respiratory symptoms are not a reason for delaying immunization. The red area and irritability after the previous immunization are normal, and the mother should have been counselled to expect this.

→ http://webarchive.nationalarchives.gov.uk/20130107105354/http:// immunisation.dh.gov.uk/gb-complete-current-edition/ ('The Green Book'; see Chapter 6. This is a key UK resource for immunization.)

3. E ★ OHCS 10th edn → pp. 188–9

This child has diabetic ketoacidosis (DKA). Fluid management has been appropriate so far, but now that she has passed urine, potassium needs to be added to her maintenance fluid, otherwise she will rapidly become hypokalaemic. Her glucose level is falling at a rate of 2.5 mmol/hour, which is about right. It should not be allowed to fall faster than 5 mmol/ hour. Once her blood glucose concentration reaches 14–17 mmol/L, you would change her IV fluid to one containing dextrose and potassium. The slight fall in her calcium level is not significant. The British Society for Paediatric Endocrinology and Diabetes has published guidelines on the management of DKA in children:

→ http://www.bsped.org.uk/clinical/docs/DKAGuideline.pdf

4. C ★ OHCS 10th edn → p. 210

A common mistake in the management of constipation is to discontinue the laxative too quickly. It should have been continued for about 6 months to allow time for the distended 'baggy' colon to return to normal, and this needs to be explained to the parents at the outset.

This girl's constipation has relapsed, and her soiling is due to overflow. The use of suppositories in young children should be avoided, if at all possible. Movicol® is an osmotic laxative (containing ethylene glycol particles).

→ http://www.nice.org.uk/guidance/CG99

5. B ★ OHCS 10th edn → p. 211

This is primary monosymptomatic nocturnal enuresis, and the boy should do well with an enuresis alarm. He should be followed up every few weeks while using it. He has not made progress after keeping a star chart for 4 weeks, so it is best not to persist with this on its own, but it could be combined with alarm treatment. Desmopressin could be used in the short term if he is not dry by the time of the cub camp. Imipramine is a second-line drug treatment because of the higher incidence of side effects. Oxybutynin would only be appropriate if there were symptoms of detrusor instability (e.g. daytime urgency and frequency). Enuresis is common.

→ http://www.nice.org.uk/guidance/CG111

6. C ★ OHCS 10th edn → p. 234

This child is moderately dehydrated due to gastroenteritis. According to the NICE traffic light system, he should have an initial trial of oral rehydration therapy (ORT), especially as he is not vomiting. The aim should be for him to drink 50 mL/kg over 4 hours. If he is not managing to drink this amount, change to nasogastric ORT. If he is vomiting, use IV fluid. If he was severely dehydrated, you would initially give 20 mL/kg IV 0.9% saline.

→ http://www.nice.org.uk/CG84

7. B ★ OHCS 10th edn → p. 137

Up to 60% of newborn infants have audible, but benign, heart murmurs in the first 24 hours of life. These are due to the increase in pulmonary blood flow that occurs after birth in association with relatively high pulmonary vascular resistance. As the pulmonary vascular resistance drops, the murmur disappears.

8. D ★ OHCS 10th edn → p. 166

This child has signs of a flitting polyarthritis—that is, arthritis affecting more than four joints that comes and goes. She also has the rash of erythema marginatum. Coupled with the recent history of a sore throat, this fits the criteria for rheumatic fever. Either two major criteria (which both of these fit) or one major and two minor criteria (fever is a minor criterion) are needed. Rheumatic fever is now less common in the UK, possibly due to the use of antibiotics to treat streptococcal throat infections. However, it is still seen in other parts of the world. It is caused by a cross-sensitivity reaction to group A *Streptococcus* in susceptible individuals.

9. A ★   OHCS 10th edn → p. 170

Appendicitis is the commonest cause of acute abdomen and should not be forgotten in children. It is rare in children under 5 years and becomes commoner with increasing age thereafter. The classic presentation is with central, colicky abdominal pain, which then spreads to the right iliac fossa and becomes constant in nature. However, the pain may not always be in a classic position, so other clues need to be looked for. Vomiting is almost universal, together with associated anorexia. Loose stool and dysuria may occur as a result of irritation from the inflamed appendix, so in a child with other symptoms, one should not automatically assume that these are due to simple gastroenteritis or a urinary tract infection.

10. B ★   OHCS 10th edn → p. 686

Barlow's test and Ortolani's test are used to check for developmental dysplasia of the hip. Barlow's test should be performed first (Barlow's = Back). Hold the thigh in one hand while stabilizing the pelvis with the other. With the leg in the midline, push back gently. If the hip is dislocat*able*, the femoral head will pop out of the acetabulum. Then perform Ortolani's test (Ortolani's = Out). Holding the leg in the same way, gently and steadily abduct the leg as far as you can, pushing up gently with your fingers on the greater trochanter. If the hip is dislocat*ed*, you will feel the femoral head pop back into the acetabulum, or the hip will simply not abduct fully.

11. D ★   OHCS 10th edn → pp. 218–19

It is important to know some of the common developmental milestones for children aged 0–5 years in all four developmental areas. In this case, development is normal, apart from the lack of language.

→ http://www.gpnotebook.co.uk/simplepage

12. C ★   OHCS 10th edn → p. 297

As the law stands, children under the age of 16 years can consent to treatment if they are judged to be Gillick-competent, but they cannot refuse treatment. A person with parental responsibility gives consent on behalf of a child under 16 years of age. As the mother is the only person with parental responsibility, it is she who should decide future treatment. However, in practice, every effort is made to help all of the parties to reach a decision together.

→ http://www.gmc-uk.org/0_18_years___English_1015.pdf_48903188. pdf

13. A ★   OHCS 10th edn → p. 136

These are symptoms of heart failure—shortness of breath and sweating, which are worse on effort (e.g. during feeding), tachypnoea, tachycardia, and hepatomegaly. This baby is also showing signs of shock. Heart failure often presents in neonates at about 4–6 weeks of age, when the pulmonary vascular resistance falls.

14. B ★   OHCS 10th edn → p. 124

Babies can lose up to 10% of their birthweight in the first week but should have regained their birthweight by 2 weeks of age. This baby has lost 150 g, which is 5.5% of 2.7 kg. Although breastfeeding was slow initially, it is now going well and should be encouraged.

15. A ★   OHCS 10th edn → p. 166

Children who have congenital heart lesions are at risk of infective endocarditis. Poor dental hygiene is a risk factor.

16. D ★

These features point to a diagnosis of rickets. This is especially common in African-Caribbean and South Asian children in the UK who are breastfed for a prolonged period. This is because dark-skinned people absorb less sunlight and there is less conversion of 7-dehydrocholesterol to previtamin D_3. This results in even lower levels of vitamin D in breast milk.

→ https://patient.info/health/vitamin-d-deficiency-including-osteomalacia-and-rickets-leaflet

17. C ★   OHCS 10th edn → p. 146

The concern here is the possibility of non-accidental injury. When thinking about the mechanism of an injury, it is vital always to take into account the child's developmental stage. In this case, consider whether a 7-month-old child is capable of climbing out of a cot.

18. E ★   OHCS 10th edn → p. 164

It is important always to reconsider a diagnosis of 'asthma' in children who do not respond to treatment and to consider referral for specialist opinion. In this case, the recurrent infections, nasal discharge, poor growth, and clubbing suggest cystic fibrosis. A sweat test is diagnostic for this and should be done. Lung function and a CT scan of the chest may be performed following diagnosis in order to obtain additional information, but the important step is making the diagnosis.

→ https://patient.info/doctor/cystic-fibrosis-pro

19. B ★   OHCS 10th edn → pp. 178–9

Nephrotic syndrome is a triad of hypoalbuminaemia, proteinuria, and oedema. It often presents with periorbital oedema just after a viral infection, and it is important to dip a urine sample to look for the proteinuria, otherwise it may be dismissed as an allergic reaction, of which angio-oedema may be a variety. The lack of blood in the urine rules out glomerulonephritis, and systemic lupus erythematosus (SLE) is rare. The presence of oedema rules out benign postural proteinuria.

20. E ★

Tension pneumothorax must always be considered in acutely ill asthmatic patients who deteriorate suddenly.

21. B ★   OHCS 10th edn → pp. 188–9

With any sick child, remember ABCDEFG—Airway, Breathing, Circulation, and Don't Ever Forget Glucose. This girl is shocked and dehydrated, and has altered consciousness and a relative hyponatraemia and hyperkalaemia caused by hyperglycaemia. The diagnosis is diabetic ketoacidosis, and a capillary blood glucose test will confirm this.

22. A ★   OHCS 10th edn → p. 158

This child is very likely to have epiglottitis. He has not been immunized so is not protected against *Haemophilus influenzae* type B, and he shows signs of upper airway obstruction. Any disturbance may cause deterioration, and an attempt to examine the throat may cause fatal respiratory arrest. Intubation is difficult due to the swollen epiglottis, and occasionally emergency tracheostomy is required. Senior anaesthetic and ear, nose, and throat (ENT) help should be summoned urgently.

23. D ★   OHCS 10th edn → p. 206

There seems to be developmental regression (at least for gross motor skills), which would not be consistent with a febrile convulsion. Other more serious diagnoses should be considered.

24. D ★   OHCS 10th edn → p. 596

This is a severe case of seborrhoeic dermatitis affecting the scalp (also known as 'cradle cap' in young children). Note the thick yellow scale and crust.

25. B ★★   OHCS 10th edn → p. 115

The benefits of breast milk far outweigh any disadvantages related to mild jaundice. Although it is not entirely clear why breastfed babies develop persistent jaundice, these babies rarely, if ever, have levels of unconjugated bilirubin high enough to cause kernicterus.

26. E ★★

The wrist X-ray shows widened, frayed, and cupped metaphyses of the radius and ulna. These changes are typical of rickets and are usually combined with osteopenia. The metaphysis is the growth plate, and it lies between the diaphysis (the shaft of the long bone) and the epiphysis (the end of the bone). This area fails to mineralize normally in the growing child, due to low vitamin D levels. The aetiology is most probably a combination of initial low vitamin D stores secondary to maternal deficiency, and ongoing low sunlight exposure.

→ http://www.bmj.com/content/340/bmj.b5664

27. B ★★   OHCS 10th edn → p. 176

This is haemolytic uraemic syndrome—low haemoglobin (anaemia), with raised urea and creatinine (uraemia). A blood film would show evidence of haemolysis. This is usually caused by verocytotoxin-producing *E. coli*, which causes an acute colitis with bloody diarrhoea. It is usually contracted after contact with animals or contaminated vegetables. After recovery from the diarrhoeal illness, the child begins to get symptoms consistent with acute kidney injury—oliguria—and anaemia—lethargy and pallor.

→ https://www.gov.uk/government/publications/vero-cytotoxin-producing-escherichia-coli-vtec-complications

28. C ★★   OHCS 10th edn → p. 201

The headache is typical of migraine. The long history and lack of any suggestive features effectively rule out a space-occupying lesion. For this reason, and because there is a clear clinical diagnosis, a CT scan is not indicated. The frequency of bad attacks (more than once a month) interfering with school justifies prophylactic treatment, and propranolol is probably most commonly used in the UK. However, it is not of proven benefit. This boy is too young to be treated with sumatriptan nasal spray (although sumatriptan can be given orally). Simple analgesia should continue to be used for headache when it occurs.

→ https://www.ichd-3.org/ (International Headache Society)

→ https://www.nice.org.uk/guidance/cg150

29. E ★★   OHCS 10th edn → p. 180

This boy is most likely to have constitutional delay in growth and puberty. As testicular enlargement is the first sign of puberty in boys, measurement of testicular volume (using an orchidometer, consisting of a string of testicle-shaped beads of different volumes) will indicate whether he has started puberty, even in the absence of other signs. If his testicular size is greater than 4 mL, you can reassure him that he has entered puberty and that the other signs and a growth spurt will follow. The pubertal growth spurt is a late event in boys. All of the other items are relevant and should be recorded.

30. E ★★   OHCS 10th edn → p. 168

All of these are tropical infections that can occur in South Asia and cause high fever. Typhoid is caused by *Salmonella enterica* serotype typhi, a Gram-negative bacillus. It is transmitted from human to human through water or food contaminated with faeces. The incubation period is usually 7–14 days, and the first phase of the illness causes increasing fever, headache, malaise, anorexia, abdominal pain, and usually diarrhoea in children. Classic features of the disease, such as rose spots, generally do not appear until the second week. Diagnosis is based on finding the bacteria on blood culture. Dengue fever is a viral infection that is transmitted via mosquito bites. The incubation period is about 4–7 days, and infection causes an acute febrile illness with headache, myalgia, and joint pain. There is a risk of developing a haemorrhagic illness as the fever subsides. Leishmaniasis is a parasitic disease that is spread by the bite of infected sand flies. It can have a very long incubation period and an abrupt or gradual onset of symptoms, which typically include fever, weight loss, and hepatosplenomegaly. Malaria is a common illness in travellers returning to the UK. It is a mosquito-borne parasitic infection caused by *Plasmodium* species. After an incubation period of 1 to 2 weeks, symptoms of fever, rigors, myalgia, headache, cough, and diarrhoea develop. Malaria is diagnosed by seeing the parasites on thick and thin blood films or by a rapid antigen test. Leptospirosis has a long incubation period of 2 to 3 weeks and is typically contracted from water that has been contaminated with the urine of animals, such as rats. The acute phase is similar to that of typhoid. However, *Leptospira* species are spirochaete bacteria.

31. A ★★   OHCS 10th edn → p. 202

This baby's presentation raises concern about the possibility of meningo-encephalitis, and ceftriaxone is a broad-spectrum antibiotic that should be started if this is suspected. The cerebrospinal fluid (CSF) picture confirms this with a raised white cell count. However, it indicates that a viral cause is likely, with a near-normal glucose level, normal protein, and mostly mononuclear cells seen. Aciclovir is an antiviral medication that can be used to treat herpes simplex, which is the most likely cause of viral encephalitis in this age group. It should be started alongside broad-spectrum antibiotics whenever viral encephalitis is thought to be a possibility. Infection with anaerobes is very unlikely in an otherwise well child, so metronidazole will offer no benefit. Intravenous dexamethasone is used at the time of giving antibiotics in bacterial meningitis, to reduce the incidence of neurological complications. Isoniazid is used to treat tuberculosis (TB). Rifampicin is sometimes used as chemoprophylaxis in cases of meningococcal meningitis.

32. D ★★★   OHCS 10th edn → p. 107

Pre-term babies lose heat very easily. Placing them immediately into a plastic bag has been shown to be most effective in conserving heat. Hypothermia is associated with a worse outcome and should be avoided.

→ http://www.resus.org.uk/pages/nls.pdf

33. A ★★★

Analgesia should not be forgotten in children who are in pain. There is well-published guidance on a step-wise approach to analgesia, starting with simple treatments and adding in further treatment. However, different analgesics are effective for different types of pain. Bony pain responds well to non-steroidal anti-inflammatory drugs (NSAIDs), and this girl is already on one of these, so another is not appropriate. In malignancy, opioids are often needed, and simple opioids such as codeine should be tried first. Diazepam and hyoscine may be adjunctive treatments in symptom control in palliative care but are not analgesics.

→ http://www.who.int/cancer/palliative/painladder/en/index.html

34. A ★★★ OHCS 10th edn → p. 132

This shows epispadias where the urethral meatus comes out on the dorsum of the penis. More common is hypospadias where the urethral meatus comes out on the ventral aspect of the penis and is often narrowed. In reconstruction of both, the foreskin may be needed, so it is vital to warn the parents not to have the child circumcised until the surgeon has made an operative assessment. Otherwise there is no increased risk of infection, and it is always better not to retract the foreskin of babies.

35. C ★★★

Drug errors are one of the commonest types of error in paediatric practice. Anyone can make an error, and the best way to improve patient safety is to improve systems and training. The parents should receive an early explanation and apology. Any such incident is serious, and you should promptly involve a senior colleague. You may think that no harm has been done, but there may be wider issues to consider, in particular the Trust's obligation under Duty of Candour guidance. Reflective portfolio entries and notification of your defence society are often appropriate but are not the most important actions.

→ http://www.nrls.npsa.nhs.uk/resources/?entryid45=65077

→ http://www.gmc-uk.org/guidance/ethical_guidance/27233.asp

36. B ★★★ OHCS 10th edn → p. 174

Note that recommendations for the investigation of UTIs in children have changed in England and Wales with the publication of the National Institute for Health and Care Excellence (NICE) guidelines. Investigation is now generally more conservative. This child is under 6 months of age, but her UTI was typical and not recurrent, and she responded to treatment within 48 hours. Therefore, she needs a renal ultrasound scan, which should be performed within 6 weeks, to look for anatomical abnormalities, but she does not require any other imaging.

→ http://www.nice.org.uk/guidance/CG54

37. E ★★★ OHCS 10th edn → pp. 156, 186

The incidence of type 2 diabetes in children is rising, although it is still far less common than type 1 diabetes. The risk is increased in children who are overweight, who have a family history of type 2 diabetes, and who are of South Asian origin. The velvety skin in this girl's axillae is characteristic of acanthosis nigricans, a finding in insulin resistance and obesity.

38. E ★★★   OHCS 10th edn → p. 118

Surfactant treatment via an endotracheal tube is the most important treatment for respiratory distress syndrome and should be given as rescue treatment as soon as the baby has been intubated. Antibiotics should also be commenced (if this has not already been done) after blood cultures have been taken, and morphine may be needed for sedation on the ventilator.

39. A ★★★   OHCS 10th edn → pp. 372–3

ADHD is part of a spectrum of hyperactive behaviour. It is characterized by lack of concentration and impulsivity, with or without hyperactivity, that pervades all areas of the child's life. It is commoner in children with learning difficulties. Autism is also part of a spectrum, characterized by impaired social interaction, impaired imagination, and a limited repertoire of interests. Dyspraxia is a developmental coordination disorder. Oppositional defiant disorder is a pattern of defiant, disobedient, and hostile behaviour.

→ http://www.nice.org.uk/guidance/CG72

40. C ★★★★   OHCS 10th edn → p. 130

This is a typical picture of oesophageal atresia, with polyhydramnios, 'blowing bubbles', respiratory distress, and inability to pass a nasogastric tube. Approximately 92% of oesophageal atresias are also associated with a tracheo-oesophageal fistula. The H-type, in which both the oesophagus and the trachea are patent but there is a small connection between them, is rare and often diagnosed later.

41. E ★★★★   OHCS 10th edn → p. 601

The combination of a sick child, an erythematous rash with exfoliation, and severe mucous membrane involvement indicates Stevens–Johnson syndrome. This is associated with some viral infections and certain drugs, including penicillins.

42. E ★★★★   OHCS 10th edn → p. 638

The MRI scan shows subependymal nodules in the left ventricle. This, combined with seizures and hypopigmented skin lesions, is strongly suggestive of tuberous sclerosis.

43. A ★★★★   OHCS 10th edn → p. 156

Catch-up growth for weight in early childhood is a risk factor for future obesity. Babies who are born small for gestational age are advised to gain weight at a slower rate than babies born at a 'normal' weight—no more than 100 g per week for the first few months, rather than 180–200 g per week.

44. D ★★★★ OHCS 10th edn → p. 136

Prostaglandin E$_2$ should be commenced because the clinical presentation is consistent with a duct-dependent congenital cardiac lesion where the duct has just closed. This means that blood can no longer flow around the body. It should cause the duct to reopen until something definitive can be done. The duct typically closes at around 48 hours of age, so a duct-dependent lesion should always be considered in babies who collapse at this age.

45. B ★★★★ OHCS 10th edn → pp. 178–9

This boy almost certainly has minimal change nephrotic syndrome (MCNS), given his age, normal blood pressure, lack of haematuria, and normal renal function and other blood tests. Around 95% of children with MCNS will respond to steroids, although most relapse at some point. The long-term outlook is good.

→ Eddy AA, Symons JM. Nephrotic syndrome in childhood. *Lancet.* 2003;**362**:629–39.

Chapter 3

Gynaecology and genitourinary medicine

Kevin Hayes

Gynaecological practices are changing constantly, with more emphasis on management in primary care, conservative, rather than surgical, management of conditions, and an increase in sub-specialization such as gynaecological oncology and urogynaecology. This chapter reflects these changes and covers the commonest areas in this interesting field.

Sexual health is a specialty in its own right. The number of cases of sexually transmitted infections are rising in the UK, despite efforts to raise awareness of safe sex, so knowledge of their presentations is important. The UK also has the highest rate of teenage pregnancy in Europe, and the Government has set targets to improve access to contraceptive advice for women. In recent years, astounding advances have been made in the treatment of human immunodeficiency virus (HIV) infection, and people with HIV can now expect to have a much better quality of life.

Although this chapter primarily focuses on diseases affecting women, we have included questions on the sexual health of men to represent the full spectrum of sexual health practice.

QUESTIONS

1. A 20-year-old woman and her 23-year-old husband have been trying to conceive for 6 months, without success. Her periods are regular. Which is the single most appropriate management at this stage? ★

A Arrange a semen analysis for the husband

B Arrange a laparoscopy and dye test for the woman

C Arrange luteal-phase progesterone levels for the woman

D Arrange referral to the assisted conception unit for *in-vitro* fertilization (IVF)

E Reassure the couple and suggest that they keep trying

2. A 55-year-old woman has hot flushes. Her last period was 2 years ago. She is keen to start hormone replacement therapy (HRT). In terms of safety of prescribing, what is the single most appropriate question to ask her before commencing HRT? ★

A Do any of your relatives have Alzheimer's disease?

B Do you know whether you have osteoporosis?

C Have any of your relatives suffered from premature menopause?

D Have you ever suffered from deep vein thrombosis?

E Have you ever suffered from depression?

3. A 14-year-old girl requests emergency contraception. She had unprotected intercourse with her 14-year-old boyfriend 2 days ago. She appears to understand the nature of emergency contraception. Which is the single most appropriate management? ★

A Advise her that she cannot have emergency contraception, as it is too long since intercourse took place

B Advise her that she is too young to be legally prescribed emergency contraception

C Prescribe emergency hormonal contraception and advise her about future contraception

D Prescribe emergency hormonal contraception only after informing her parents

E Prescribe emergency hormonal contraception only after informing social services

4. A 31-year-old woman has vulval soreness and recurrent white vaginal discharge. Microscopy shows the presence of hyphae. Which is the single most appropriate treatment option? ★

A Clindamycin

B Clotrimazole

C Doxycycline

D Erythromycin

E Metronidazole

5. A 35-year-old woman who is taking Cerazette® (a progestogen-only contraceptive pill) has a chest infection and is prescribed amoxicillin. Which single piece of advice should be given about her contraception? ★

A No additional contraceptive precautions are required

B Use additional precautions for the duration of the antibiotic course

C Use additional precautions for the duration of the antibiotic course and for 2 days after the end of the course

D Use additional precautions for the duration of the antibiotic course and for 7 days after the end of the course

E Use additional precautions for the remainder of the current packet of Cerazette®

6. A 32-year-old woman has increasing white vaginal discharge. She is 7 weeks pregnant. Her *Chlamydia* swab is positive. All other tests are normal. Which is the single most appropriate treatment? ★

A Amoxicillin

B Clindamycin

C Doxycycline

D Erythromycin

E Metronidazole

7. A 42-year-old woman has frequency, urgency, and urge incontin-ence. Examination is unremarkable and a midstream specimen of urine is sterile. She is treated empirically for detrusor overactivity with oxybutynin. What is the principal mechanism of action for this drug? ★

A Anti-adrenergic

B Anti-GABAergic

C Anti-muscarinic

D Anti-nicotinic

E Anti-serotonergic

8. A 60-year-old woman is recovering post-operatively following a vaginal hysterectomy and anterior vaginal repair. She has had voiding difficulty and has been catheterized for 3 days. A catheter specimen of urine is taken due to a low-grade pyrexia, and it confirms the presence of a urinary tract infection (UTI). Which single organism is most likely to be causative? ★

A *Escherichia coli*

B *Klebsiella pneumoniae*

C *Proteus* species

D *Pseudomonas* species

E *Staphylococcus epidermidis*

9. A 24-year-old woman has had an abnormal vaginal discharge for the past week. It is off-white and non-itchy, with an offensive odour. She has had one sexual partner in the last 8 months, and he has no symptoms. There is an off-white vaginal discharge pooling in the posterior fornix, with no inflammation of the vulva or vagina. Which is the single most likely finding on a Gram-stained sample of the vaginal discharge? ★

A Gram-negative intracellular diplococci

B Gram-positive and Gram-negative mixed bacteria

C Numerous lactobacilli

D Polymorphonuclear leucocytes

E Yeast cells with hyphae

10. A 14-year-old girl has been sexually active for 6 months and seeks sexual health advice. She has a regular partner and has no symptoms. She is very anxious that her mother does not find out that she is sexually active, and she wants reassurance that her confidentiality will be maintained. In which single situation might breaching her confidentiality be justified? ★

A She is found to have a sexually transmitted infection

B She is in a sexually abusive relationship

C She requests a prescription for the oral contraceptive pill

D She requests a termination of pregnancy

E None of the above, as she has an absolute right to confidentiality

11. A 25-year-old woman has her first routine cervical cytology test as part of the NHS Cervical Screening Programme. This shows 'mild dyskaryosis' and her High Risk human papillomavirus (HPV) test is positive. She attends the colposcopy clinic and has a biopsy-proven diagnosis of cervical intraepithelial neoplasia (CIN) 1. She has a body mass index (BMI) of 30 kg/m² and uses a progestogen-only oral contraceptive pill. She smokes 15 cigarettes daily and drinks approximately 25 units of alcohol per week. She wants to know if there is anything she can do that might help to reverse the abnormality. Which single action that she can be advised about is most likely to increase the chances of spontaneous resolution of her cervical abnormality? ★

A Get vaccinated against HPV infection

B Give up smoking cigarettes

C Reduce alcohol consumption

D Reduce BMI

E Switch to an alternative contraceptive pill

12. A 24-year-old woman requests post-coital contraception. Her condom broke 36 hours ago, on day 7 of a regular 29-day cycle. She is undecided about future contraceptive use. A pregnancy test is negative. Which is the single most effective form of post-coital contraception for her? ★

A A combined oral oestrogen/progestogen pill

B A progestogen-only pill

C Insertion of a copper-containing intrauterine device (IUD)

D Insertion of a progestogen-containing intrauterine system (IUS)

E No post-coital contraception is required

13. A 27-year-old man has had mild dysuria for 1 week. He has been having sex with his current girlfriend for 4 weeks, occasionally using condoms. She has no symptoms. He last had sex with his previous female partner 3 months ago. There is a slight mucoid discharge at the urethral meatus. Which single organism is the most likely cause? ★

A Chlamydia trachomatis

B Mycoplasma hominis

C Neisseria gonorrhoeae

D Trichomonas vaginalis

E Ureaplasma urealyticum

14. A 32-year-old man has a history of weight loss and general malaise. He takes a human immunodeficiency virus (HIV) test. The result is positive and his CD4+ count is 180×10^6/L (12%) (normal range is 450–1600×10^6/L). He is otherwise well. He does not feel ready to start antiretroviral therapy straight away but is keen to stay well in the interim. For which single organism should he be offered primary prophylaxis? ★

A *Cryptococcus neoformans*

B *Mycobacterium avium intracellulare*

C *Mycobacterium tuberculosis*

D *Pneumocystis jirovecii*

E *Toxoplasma gondii*

15. A 19-year-old woman has had pain in her vulval area for 4 days. A photograph of the vulval lesion is shown in Figure 3.1 (see Colour Plate section). Which is the single most likely diagnosis? ★

A Behçet's disease

B Genital herpes

C Lichen sclerosis

D Syphilitic ulcer

E Vulval cancer

16. A 19-year-old woman has had pain in her vulval area for 4 days. A photograph of the vulval lesion is shown in Figure 3.1 (see Colour Plate section). Which is the single most appropriate initial management? ★ ★

A Perform a vulval biopsy

B Prescribe oral aciclovir

C Prescribe oral azithromycin

D Prescribe oral prednisolone

E Prescribe topical clobetasol (Dermovate®)

17. A 29-year-old man from South Africa has collapsed at work. An eyewitness gives a clear description of a convulsion. The man is drowsy, barely rousable, and unable to communicate. His wife states that she fears he may be human immunodeficiency virus (HIV)-positive. His breathing becomes erratic, and artificial ventilation is being considered. In which single situation should an HIV test be carried out, given that he is unable to give informed consent? ★ ★

A At the request of his wife, as next of kin

B If knowledge of his HIV status would benefit his care

C Prior to admitting him to the intensive therapy unit

D Prior to any invasive procedure being performed

E Prior to making the decision to ventilate

18. A 23-year-old woman has a large, 20-week-sized cystic mass on her ovary. She undergoes laparotomy and oophorectomy, and histology confirms that this is a benign mucinous cystadenoma. Which is the single most likely ovarian tissue of origin for this type of cyst? ★ ★

A Epithelial

B Follicular

C Germ cell

D Sex cord

E Stromal

19. A 22-year-old woman who is struggling to conceive has the following hormone profile, taken on day 6 of her cycle:

- luteinizing hormone (LH): 12 IU/mL (normal pre-menopausal range, 3–13 IU/mL)
- follicle-stimulating hormone (FSH): 4 IU/mL (normal range, 3–20 IU/mL)
- testosterone: 18 ng/dL (normal range, 6–86 ng/dL).

An ultrasound scan shows numerous peripheral ovarian follicles. Which single set of symptoms is she most likely to have? ★ ★

A Amenorrhoea and infertility

B Amenorrhoea and pelvic pain

C Oligomenorrhoea and facial hair

D Oligomenorrhoea and pelvic pain

E Oligomenorrhoea and temporal headaches

20. A 24-year-old man who has sex with men has read on the Internet that his sexual orientation puts him at risk of hepatitis B virus (HBV) infection. He is interested in being immunized. His hepatitis status results are as follows:

- hepatitis B virus surface antigen (HBsAg) negative
- hepatitis B virus core antibody (HBcAb) positive
- hepatitis B virus surface antibody (HBsAb) negative
- hepatitis B virus e antigen (HBeAg) negative.

Which is the single most appropriate advice regarding his results and proposed immunization? ★★

A He has evidence of previous exposure to HBV and is a 'high-risk' carrier; immunization will not help

B He has evidence of previous exposure to HBV and is a 'low-risk' carrier; immunization will not help

C He has evidence of previous exposure to HBV, with a partial immune response; immunization is unlikely to help

D He has evidence of previous exposure to HBV, with an appropriate immune response; immunization is unnecessary

E He has no evidence of previous exposure to HBV and should proceed with immunization as planned

21. A 16-year-old girl has had painful periods for 6 months. Her periods are regular and last 3 days. She misses a couple of days of school every month due to the pain. She is not sexually active. Which is the single most appropriate initial management? ★★

A Gonadotrophin-releasing hormone analogues

B Intrauterine system (Mirena®)

C Mefenamic acid

D Progesterone-only oral contraceptive pill

E Tranexamic acid

22. A 26-year-old woman with no children has had amenorrhoea for 6 weeks and has some pelvic discomfort. Her pregnancy test is positive. Her pulse rate is 68 bpm, and her blood pressure is 110/80 mmHg. An ultrasound scan shows an empty uterus, with normal adnexae. Her serum β-human chorionic gonadotrophin (β-HCG) level is 950 mIU/mL. Which is the single most appropriate next step in management? ★★

A Arrange for a laparoscopy

B Arrange for a laparotomy

C Repeat the β-HCG test after 48 hours

D Repeat the ultrasound scan and β-HCG test after 48 hours

E Repeat the ultrasound scan after 48 hours

23. A 30-year-old nurse sustained a significant needle-stick injury during her last shift, 36 hours ago. The patient (i.e. 'donor') involved is human immunodeficiency virus (HIV)-positive. He is taking antiretroviral therapy, and his last viral load was 1000 copies/mL (acceptable load is <5000 copies/mL). He is hepatitis B virus-immune and negative for hepatitis C virus. The nurse also had unprotected sex earlier in her current menstrual cycle, and there is a possibility that she may be pregnant. Which is the single most appropriate advice regarding HIV post-exposure prophylaxis (PEP)? ★ ★

A It is already too late for her to start taking PEP

B PEP is contraindicated because of the possibility that she is pregnant

C She does not need PEP, as the patient's viral load is so low

D She should start PEP without further delay

E The risks associated with PEP are higher than the risk of acquiring HIV

24. A 42-year-old man attends a genitourinary medicine clinic and asks for a routine check for sexually transmitted infections. He has no symptoms and no abnormal clinical findings. Serological tests for syphilis show:

- rapid plasma reagin (RPR) positive at a titre of 1:64
- *Treponema pallidum* particle agglutination (TPPA) assay positive
- fluorescent treponemal antibody absorption test (FTA-ABS) positive.

The same tests were negative 18 months ago. Which single stage of syphilis can be diagnosed? ★ ★

A Early latent

B Late latent

C Primary

D Secondary

E Tertiary

25. A 22-year-old woman is 6–8 weeks pregnant and is brought into the Emergency Department in cardiac arrest. No other medical information about her is available. Which is the single most likely cause of her cardiac arrest in early pregnancy? ★ ★

A Miscarriage bleeding

B Pre-existing cardiac disease

C Pulmonary embolus

D Ruptured ectopic pregnancy

E Sepsis following termination of pregnancy

26. A 22-year-old woman has an acute onset of right iliac fossa pain, but no vomiting. She has marked tenderness to palpation in the right iliac fossa. There is no rebound tenderness and some voluntary guarding. Her temperature is 37.2°C, her pulse rate 80 bpm, and her blood pressure 115/80 mmHg. Her pregnancy test is negative. An ultrasound scan shows a 7-cm right-sided haemorrhagic ovarian cyst with no free fluid. Which is the single most appropriate initial management? ★★★

A Admit her with a view to conservative management

B Allow her to go home, with advice to come back if the pain worsens

C Perform an immediate laparoscopy in case the diagnosis is torsion

D Refer to the surgeons to rule out appendicitis

E Request a computed tomography (CT) scan to confirm the diagnosis

27. A 70-year-old woman has had vulval itching and discomfort for 12 months. There is widespread erythema on both labia minora, extending onto the majora and involving the fourchette. There are no ulcers and there is no inguinal lymphadenopathy. Which is the single most appropriate initial management? ★★★

A Empirical treatment with potent corticosteroid ointment

B Immediate punch biopsy to exclude cancer

C Referral to the sexual health clinic to rule out a sexually transmitted infection

D Treatment with oestrogen cream for atrophy

E Vulval excision to treat the affected area

28. A 24-year-old woman has dysmenorrhoea and deep dyspareunia. A transvaginal ultrasound scan shows a 4-cm endometrioma on the left ovary. The patient wants relief of her pain symptoms. She has also been trying to conceive for over 12 months. Which is the single most appropriate treatment to use? ★★★

A Combined oral contraceptive pill

B Danazol

C Gonadotrophin-releasing hormone analogues

D Laparoscopic surgery

E Medroxyprogesterone acetate (Provera®)

29. A previously well 67-year-old woman has abdominal distension, a large irregular pelvic mass, and ascites. An ultrasound scan, a computed tomography (CT) scan, and a raised CA125 confirm a likely ovarian carcinoma. Which is the single most appropriate first-line management? ★ ★ ★

A External beam radiotherapy

B High-dose progestogen therapy

C Hysterectomy, bilateral oophorectomy, omentectomy, and debulking

D Symptomatic palliative care

E Vincristine-containing chemotherapy

ANSWERS

1. E ★   OHCS 10th edn → p. 292

Normal healthy couples can take up to a year to conceive, so investigations are not normally started until after 1 year of regular attempts to conceive.

2. D ★   OHCS 10th edn → p. 256

Overall, HRT doubles the risk of venous thromboembolism, so other risk factors need to be considered. HRT helps to reduce the risk of fractures in osteoporosis. There is no association with Alzheimer's disease; in fact, HRT may be protective. In some women, symptoms of depression may occur with some forms of HRT, but this would not be a contraindication.

→ https://www.nice.org.uk/guidance/ng23

3. C ★   OHCS 10th edn → pp. 297, 299

The girl appears to be Gillick-competent, as she understands the nature of the treatment. Therefore, she should be prescribed emergency contraception, like any other patient. Emergency contraception can be given up to 72 hours after unprotected sex. Thought must be given to ongoing contraception to avoid further incidents.

→ http://www.nhs.uk/Livewell/Sexandyoungpeople/Pages/Willthey tellmyparents.aspx

4. B ★   OHCS 10th edn → p. 284

Hyphae indicate the presence of *Candida* or 'thrush'. Antibiotics are not an appropriate treatment for a fungal infection. Clotrimazole is an antifungal topical treatment.

5. A ★   OHCS 10th edn → pp. 300–3

Most people remember that there is some interaction between the combined oral contraceptive pill and antibiotics. In truth, the evidence is slight, but the official advice to women taking the combined oral contraceptive pill is to use additional contraceptive methods for the duration of the course and for 7 oral contraceptive pill-taking days afterwards (i.e. the pill-free week does not 'count', so if a pill-free week is coming up, the woman might want to run two packets together). However, this rule does not apply to progestogen-only contraceptive pills, such as Cerazette®, and the woman should continue to take this continuously at the same time every day.

→ http://www.nhs.uk/Conditions/contraception-guide/Pages/combined-contraceptive-pill.aspx

6. D ★   OHCS 10th edn → p. 285

Amoxicillin, clindamycin, and metronidazole are ineffective against *Chlamydia*, and doxycycline is contraindicated in pregnancy.

7. C ★   OHCS 10th edn → p. 307

Detrusor contraction is activated via muscarinic cholinergic receptors, and oxybutynin is a direct anti-muscarinic agent. Serotonin and nor-adrenaline (norepinephrine) are important for sympathetic activation, which reduces detrusor activity intrinsically. There are no nicotinic or GABAergic receptors in the bladder.

8. A ★

E. coli is by far the commonest cause of sporadic or catheter-related urinary tract infection. *Pseudomonas* species are usually only associated with prolonged catheterization, and *S. epidermidis* is usually a contaminant.

9. B ★   OHCS 10th edn → p. 284

This is a description of bacterial vaginosis, which is caused by an altered vaginal flora and overgrowth of a number of different microorganisms, which may show up on Gram staining.

10. B ★   OHCS 10th edn → p. 297

The doctor has to judge whether the girl is Gillick-competent, and if she is, she can consent to treatment herself. However, if she is thought to be the victim of any kind of sexual abuse and/or coercion, safeguarding rules trump her right of confidentiality, and the doctor has a duty of care to at least seek advice—for example, from the local named doctor for safeguarding children. The General Medical Council (GMC) gives guidance on this, which should be read.

→ http://www.gmc-uk.org/guidance/ethical_guidance/confidentiality

11. B ★   OHCS 10th edn → pp. 272–3

All of these are protective against cervical changes. HPV vaccination has now been introduced into the UK and will help to prevent changes from occurring. However, in this case, in which the changes are already present, it will not be effective. The evidence shows that smoking is the most important risk factor in women who show mild change.

12. C ★   OHCS 10th edn → p. 299

Combined oral contraceptive pills are no longer used for post-coital contraception. There is no efficacy advantage, and they have more side effects than Levonelle® (a progestogen-only pill). Levonelle® may be an option. However, it does not offer the additional benefit of an ongoing method of contraception, and there is also a recognized failure rate. An IUD is always the most effective form of post-coital contraception for anyone, but in this case it has the added advantage of providing ongoing contraception. Mirena® coils are not used for post-coital contraception.

13. **A** ★

Chlamydia is the commonest sexually transmitted infection in the UK. Around 50% of men have no symptoms, but those that do may have dysuria, epididymo-orchitis, clear penile discharge, and low-grade fever.

14. **D** ★

P. jirovecii (previously known as *Pneumocystis carinii*) can cause severe pneumonia (*P. carinii* pneumonia or PCP) in immunocompromised individuals. The risk increases when the CD4+ count falls below 200 × 10^6/L, especially if the viral load is detectable. Therefore, measures are taken to try to prevent this with antibiotic prophylaxis. It has been standard practice for many years to offer HIV patients with a CD4+ count of less than 200 × 10^6/L primary prophylaxis against *Pneumocystis*. Without prophylactic therapy, *Pneumocystis* is the single most likely serious or life-threatening opportunistic infection they will develop. Patients can develop *C. neoformans* infection, but it is much less common, and primary prophylaxis is not given, although secondary prophylaxis would be continued in those who do develop it until their CD4+ count rises in response to therapy. *M. avium intracellulare* is unlikely to be a problem with a CD4+ count of more than 100/μL, and primary prophylaxis is not routinely given. *M. tuberculosis* can of course affect any patient, regardless of the CD4+ count, but primary prophylaxis is not given. *T. gondii* is unlikely to be a problem with a CD4+ count of more than 50/μL, so primary prophylaxis would not be given in this case.

15. **B** ★   OHCS 10th edn → p. 268

Genital herpes causes multiple painful sores on the vulva and may also cause lymphadenopathy and flu-like symptoms. It is the only common cause of genital ulceration in this age group. Behçet's syndrome can cause genital ulceration but is rare. Lichen sclerosus causes white, atrophic-looking areas and usually occurs in older women. Syphilitic chancres are usually single and ulcerated.

16. **B** ★★   OHCS 10th edn → p. 268

This is herpes simplex virus infection, so antiviral treatment is required.

17. **B** ★★

General principles of consent mean that the patient is the only person capable of giving consent for any investigation or treatment. If the medical information may guide his treatment (e.g. determining which drugs to start), investigations can be performed when he is unable to give consent. This would be acting in the patient's best interests. However, this is rarely straightforward, and the General Medical Council (GMC) guidance on consent should be read. Universal precautions mean that full infection control precautions should be taken for *all* patients, regardless of whether they are known to be HIV-positive or not.

→ http://www.gmc-uk.org/guidance/ethical_guidance/consent_guidance_scope_of_treatment_in_emergencies.asp

18. A ★★ OHCS 10th edn → p. 281

Adenomata, by definition, are derived from the ovarian glandular epithelium. They can produce serous or mucinous cystadenomas.

19. C ★★ OHCS 10th edn → p. 252

A reversed LH:FSH ratio of around 3:1 and numerous small peripheral follicles in the ovaries are characteristic of polycystic ovary syndrome (PCOS). This is sometimes seen, but the most sensitive biochemical test for PCOS is a high free androgen index (testosterone:sex hormone-binding globulin ratio). The symptoms of this include reduced periods, reduced fertility, hirsutism, acne, and weight gain.

20. C ★★

This patient has detectable HBcAb. The only way that an individual can develop core antibody is in response to HBV infection. There is no core antigen in the vaccine. However, the patient is HBsAg-negative and HBeAg-negative, so he is not a chronic virus carrier. Unfortunately, he has not developed any HBsAb, which is the antibody that confers protective immunity (and what the vaccine aims to produce). There is some controversy as to whether vaccinating patients with a blunted response to previous HBV infection achieves anything (if the infection did not result in immunity, the vaccine is unlikely to do any better). However, there is no evidence base for it.

21. C ★★ OHCS 10th edn → p. 250

Mefenamic acid is effective for the management of period pain and can be taken around the time of the period only. Tranexamic acid has some pain-relieving properties but is more effective for the treatment of heavy periods. An intrauterine system (IUS) would be one option, but as the patient is not sexually active, this would not be the first-line management. The progesterone-only pill may well lighten periods but does not necessarily relieve the pain. Gonadotrophin-releasing hormone analogues have no role.

22. C ★★ OHCS 10th edn → pp. 262–3

This is a pregnancy of unknown location. The β-HCG level is only slightly lower than 1000 mIU/mL, and we need to know what is happening with the trophoblastic activity. The woman is clinically well and not shocked, so urgent treatment is not needed. β-HCG levels normally double over 48 hours, so a repeat test will help to decide if this is likely to be a normal pregnancy, a possible ectopic pregnancy, or a failing one.

23. D ★★

If the donor in a needle-stick injury is at high risk for blood-borne viruses, PEP should be started straight away until confirmatory testing can be done. Delays reduce the effectiveness. Many antiretroviral drugs are safe in pregnancy. Indeed, pregnant HIV-positive women are advised to take antiretroviral drugs to reduce the risk of HIV transmission to the fetus.

→ http://www.patient.info/doctor/hiv-post-exposure-prophylaxis

→ http://www.bhiva.org/documents/Guidelines/PEPSE/PEPSE2011.pdf

24. A ★★

There are four stages of syphilis:

- primary: characterized by painless ulcers, called chancres, at the site of infection. They may not be noticed. Chancres occur about 3 weeks after infection
- secondary: occurs 2–10 weeks after the chancres appear. Symptoms include a rash, mouth ulcers, lymphadenopathy, fever, and myalgia
- latent: occurs months to years after the initial infection if it goes untreated and it is usually asymptomatic, but the infection remains in the body
- tertiary: occurs years after the initial infection in a minority of people and can affect almost any part of the body.

Testing for syphilis can be complex because of the different stages. However, in an individual who is asymptomatic but has positive serological tests, this implies that the infection is latent. If the patient is known to have acquired the infection within the last 2 years, it is early latent. In this case, we can be completely confident that the infection is less than 2 years old, because we are told that the syphilis serology was negative 18 months ago.

25. D ★★   OHCS 10th edn → pp. 262–3

The commonest cause of arrest and death in early pregnancy is hypovolaemia due to a ruptured ectopic pregnancy, and it is the first consideration in a collapsed patient in early pregnancy. Heavy vaginal bleeding rarely presents in an arrest, as help tends to be sought early for visible bleeding. The risk of a pulmonary embolus is raised throughout pregnancy, but the most severe morbidity and mortality occur in later trimesters or postpartum, and both sepsis due to termination and pre-existing cardiac conditions are fortunately rare.

→ http://www.oaa-anaes.ac.uk/UI/Content/

26. A ★★★   OHCS 10th edn → p. 280

A patient with marked tenderness should not be allowed home. The history, examination, and ultrasound scan findings are highly suggestive and commensurate with a haemorrhagic cyst accident, which should be managed conservatively. The absence of vomiting, peritonism, and pyrexia makes torsion and appendicitis unlikely, and there is no need to refer the patient to the surgeons at this stage, as the diagnosis is basically straightforward. Therefore, no further imaging is required at this stage.

27. A ★★★ OHCS 10th edn → p. 266

This is likely to be lichen sclerosus et atrophicus, a poorly understood inflammatory condition. It responds well to potent corticosteroid ointment, and a biopsy is indicated if there is no response to treatment or if an actual suspicious lesion, such as an ulcer, is present. Oestrogen cream is only effective for pure atrophy, and the likelihood of a sexually transmitted infection in a 70-year-old is very small. Excision is reserved for neoplastic conditions.

28. D ★★★ OHCS 10th edn → p. 288

All of the medical treatments listed are effective for pain, although there is increasing evidence that surgery gives the best results overall. Endometriomata tend to respond poorly to medical treatment and usually require excision. Only surgical treatment has been demonstrated to improve subsequent fertility which is relevant to this case.

29. C ★★★ OHCS 10th edn → p. 283

Primary pelvic clearance and tumour debulking are the mainstays of ovarian cancer treatment initially. Neoadjuvant chemotherapy is a reasonable option in some women but involves the use of carboplatin and paclitaxel, not vincristine. Hormonal treatment and radiotherapy have little or no place in ovarian cancer treatment, and palliative care is for women with terminal disease who have not responded to surgery and chemotherapy.

Psychiatry

Isabel McMullen

Mental health problems are estimated to affect one in four people each year in the UK, making mental illness one of the commonest presentations to GP surgeries, outpatient clinics, and Emergency Departments. Yet many doctors and medical students feel uncertain about how to approach patients with a psychiatric disorder.

The key to becoming a good psychiatrist lies in the clinical interview. There are few physical signs or investigations that allow doctors to diagnose psychiatric illness, so a detailed history and mental state examination are important. As a psychiatrist, you are in the privileged position of having patients tell you their personal stories, and the skill is in listening attentively and asking relevant questions to help to clarify parts of the story. The best way to practise these techniques is to watch experienced clinicians at work and to interview patients yourself.

Obviously diagnosis is important, so you need to be aware of the types of symptoms that fit with each type of disorder, as well as the medical conditions that may mimic psychiatric illness. Investigations may be necessary to rule out other diseases, and you need to be able to request these appropriately. Psychiatrists have access to a range of treatments—medical (e.g. antidepressants), psychological (e.g. cognitive behavioural therapy), and physical (e.g. electroconvulsive therapy)—and you need to know which ones to recommend. Most of these treatments are delivered in conjunction with the multidisciplinary team, so you should be clear about the roles of each team member.

Finally, there is overlap between psychiatry and the law, which can raise interesting ethical issues. It is sometimes necessary to treat a person against their will, for the safety of that person or others, so you need to know about mental health law. Psychiatrists are also often requested to provide a second opinion in difficult capacity assessments.

QUESTIONS

1. A 53-year-old builder has injured his arm and is admitted to the ward. Late one night, he becomes aggressive, shouting at the nurses and other patients, wanting to leave the ward, and saying that he can see ants running all over the walls. Which is the single most likely cause of these symptoms? ★

A Abnormal reaction to analgesic medication

B Alcohol withdrawal

C Dissocial personality disorder

D Head injury

E Past history of schizophrenia

2. A 20-year-old woman took 40 paracetamol tablets 9 hours ago. Which is the single most appropriate emergency treatment? ★

A Activated charcoal

B Diazepam

C Flumazenil

D *N*-acetylcysteine

E Naloxone

3. A 34-year-old woman has severe abdominal pain and blood in her stool. Abdominal and pelvic examinations are normal, except for multiple surgical scars over the abdomen, consistent with laparoscopies and an appendicectomy. She provides stool samples obtained at home that contain blood but has not managed to produce one in hospital. Blood and urine investigations are normal, but she insists on further investigation and does not want to leave hospital. Which is the single most likely diagnosis? ★

A Delusional disorder

B Hypochondriacal disorder

C Malingering

D Mild–moderate depressive episode

E Munchausen syndrome

4. A 25-year-old man is disorientated and has slurred speech and respiratory depression. He also has miosis. Which is the single most likely cause? ★

A Alcohol abuse

B Carbon monoxide (CO) poisoning

C Opioid abuse

D Paracetamol overdose

E Salicylate overdose

5. A 36-year-old man goes to a plastic surgeon insisting on surgery, stating that his nose is too large and crooked. He says that people stare at him when he goes out, so he prefers not to leave the house. He attributes his recent job loss to his 'deformed nose'. He wears make-up to camouflage it but would like surgery to correct what appears to be a normal nose. Which is the single most likely diagnosis? ★

A Body dysmorphic disorder

B Hypochondriasis

C Mild–moderate depressive episode

D Obsessive–compulsive disorder

E Social phobia

6. A 61-year-old man attends his general practitioner (GP) at the request of his wife, who thinks he is drinking too much alcohol. Which single factor is a sign of alcohol dependence? ★

A A wide repertoire of alcoholic drinks

B Decreased alcohol tolerance

C Drinking 28 units of alcohol or more a week

D Drinking despite evidence of its harm to job and family

E Drinking until late in the evening

7. A 20-year-old man has a first episode of psychosis. Your consultant asks you to prescribe an atypical (or second-generation) antipsychotic. Which single drug should be prescribed? ★

A Chlorpromazine

B Haloperidol

C Lorazepam

D Mirtazapine

E Olanzapine

8. A 64-year-old man is recovering after a myocardial infarction (MI). His recovery is slowed by poor sleep, loss of appetite, lack of motivation, and feelings of hopelessness. Your consultant believes that he is depressed and asks you to commence antidepressant treatment. He has no other medical history. Which would be the single most appropriate class of drug to prescribe? ★

A Benzodiazepine

B Monoamine oxidase inhibitor (MAOI)

C Selective serotonin reuptake inhibitor (SSRI)

D Serotonin and noradrenaline (norepinephrine) reuptake inhibitor

E Tricyclic antidepressant

9. A 52-year-old woman has low mood, tiredness, and weight gain, with decreased appetite. She is tearful and overweight, with dry skin and thin hair. Which is the single most useful test to aid diagnosis? ★

A Chest X-ray

B Electrocardiogram (ECG)

C Full blood count

D Thyroid function tests

E Urea and electrolytes

10. A 35-year-old woman suddenly starts to feel dizzy and short of breath, with chest pains and a tingling sensation in her fingers. These symptoms worsen until she feels as if she is about to die. The episode lasts for about 10 minutes before resolving completely. Which is the single most likely diagnosis? ★

A Acute asthma

B Myocardial infarction

C Panic attack

D Temporal lobe epilepsy

E Transient ischaemic attack

11. A 36-year-old woman is 36 weeks pregnant with twins in England. She has obsessive–compulsive disorder. She is scheduled to have an elective Caesarean section for the delivery of her twins, due to complications in her last delivery and pre-eclampsia in this pregnancy. She has already consented to the operation. She has now become agitated and anxious and is refusing to cooperate, saying that she does not want to have the operation and wants to go home. Which is the single most appropriate course of action? ★

A Arrange emergency detention under the Mental Health Act 2007 (England and Wales), as her health depends on her being treated

B Assess her capacity to consent, and discuss the situation with a senior doctor

C Detain her for treatment, as she has a mental disorder as defined by the Mental Health Act 2007 (England and Wales)

D Prescribe sedative medication, and advise the nurses to call when she is less agitated

E Tell the nurses to reassure her and carry on, as she has previously consented to the operation

12. A 44-year-old woman has taken an overdose of 20 paracetamol tablets. Which single factor indicates the highest risk of her going on to complete suicide? ★

A Having a psychotic illness

B Living with a partner

C Taking alcohol with the overdose

D Taking more than 50 tablets as an overdose

E Writing a suicide note before taking the overdose

13. A 58-year-old woman has gastritis. Her general practitioner (GP) is concerned about her possible heavy use of alcohol and arranges some screening questionnaires and blood tests. Which single result would indicate possible problem drinking or hazardous drinking? ★

A A decreased mean corpuscular volume (MCV)

B A low level of gamma-glutamyl transpeptidase (GGT)

C A score of 5 on the Alcohol Use Disorders Identification Test (AUDIT)

D One positive response on the CAGE questionnaire

E Raised urate levels

14. A 34-year-old man is brought to the Emergency Department by the police. He is agitated and elated. His blood pressure is 140/90 mmHg, his pulse rate 120 bpm, and his pupils dilated. Which single substance is he most likely to have been using? ★

A Cocaine

B Heroin

C Organic solvents

D Oxazepam

E Psilocybin

15. A 68-year-old man has a prominent impairment of recent memory with intact immediate recall. He has no evidence of generalized cognitive impairment and no impairment in his level of consciousness. Which is the single most likely diagnosis? ★

A Alzheimer's disease

B Delirium

C Korsakoff's syndrome

D Normal-pressure hydrocephalus

E Post-ictal state

16. A 74-year-old woman has bowel cancer being treated in England. The surgeons say that she requires surgery, which is potentially curative, and that without it she will die. The woman is refusing any surgical intervention. She had postnatal depression 42 years ago but is not currently suffering from any mental illness. Her present Mini-Mental State Examination (MMSE) score is 29/30. She knows about her diagnosis, believes that it applies to her, understands the risks and benefits of the proposed surgery, and is able to retain the information. Which is the single most appropriate course of action? ★

A Detain her under a section of the Mental Health Act 2007 (England and Wales) and perform the operation

B Discharge her from hospital

C Obtain a second opinion, and if that professional considers that the woman has capacity, comply with her wishes

D Restrain her under common law, and perform the operation

E Use the Mental Capacity Act 2005 (England and Wales) to perform the operation

17. A 40-year-old woman is having intrusive and persistent thoughts that she is a 'dirty prostitute'. She recognizes that her thoughts are silly but nevertheless feels ashamed of them. Although these thoughts get her down, she still enjoys life. Which is the single most likely diagnosis? ★

A Depressive disorder

B Generalized anxiety disorder

C Obsessive–compulsive disorder

D Psychotic episode

E Schizophrenia

18. A 28-year-old man is found in an alleyway in a semi-conscious state. He has a respiratory rate of 6 breaths/minute, a pulse rate of 50 bpm, and pinpoint pupils. Which is the single most appropriate drug to give? ★

A Clonidine

B Methadone

C Naloxone

D Naltrexone

E Thiamine

19. An 82-year-old man is forgetful, gets lost when he is out, and has difficulty finding his way home. On occasion, he puts his keys in the microwave, and he does not appear to know how to use it to cook food. His memory problems seemed to get markedly worse around the time when he was admitted to hospital with a stroke 2 years ago, and again earlier this year when he could not speak for several minutes. His speech has since recovered. Which is the single most likely diagnosis? ★

A Alzheimer's disease

B Fronto-temporal dementia

C Lewy body dementia

D Normal ageing

E Vascular dementia

20. A 28-year-old woman has low mood and loss of appetite. She is still coping at work but lacks energy and feels that her concentration is not as good as before. Her sleep is normal, and she enjoys spending time with her friends. She has never had any ideas of self-harm or suicide. Which is the single most appropriate course of action? ★

A Ask her to keep a mood diary and return to see you in 2 weeks' time

B Prescribe citalopram, and see her again in 2 weeks' time

C Prescribe moclobemide, and see her again in 4 weeks' time

D Refer her for cognitive behavioural therapy

E Tell her not to worry and that it is normal to feel like this

21. A 29-year-old woman has recently been diagnosed as having generalized anxiety disorder. Which is the single best initial approach to management? ★

A Advise her to keep a diary of when she feels anxious

B Explain the condition to her, writing down the essential points

C Give her a standard information leaflet

D Provide her with information on the medication that can be used

E Recommend a self-help book

22. A 48-year-old man with alcohol dependence has been found wandering in the street. He has some clouding of consciousness, nystagmus, and ophthalmoplegia. Which is the single most appropriate medication to administer initially? ★

A Acamprosate

B Disulfiram

C Metoclopramide

D Naloxone

E Thiamine

23. A 30-year-old woman with panic disorder has been treated with cognitive behavioural therapy, which has only partially helped her symptoms. She requests further treatment and is prescribed citalopram. Which is the single most likely side-effect profile she should be warned about? ★

A Confusion and memory problems

B Drowsiness, palpitations, and postural hypotension

C Dry mouth, blurred vision, and constipation

D Nausea, gastrointestinal upset, restlessness, and insomnia

E Weight gain

24. A 28-year-old man who has recently been diagnosed with paranoid schizophrenia is started on risperidone. Which single common potential side-effect should he be advised about? ★

A Feeling more alert

B Gynaecomastia

C Hirsutism

D Improved sexual performance

E Weight loss

25. A 67-year-old man was diagnosed with dementia a year ago. He has previously been advised, both verbally and in writing, to inform the Driver and Vehicle Licensing Agency (DVLA) of his diagnosis. He says that he has not taken this advice, as he needs his car to get to the shops and to see his friends. The Mini-Mental State Examination (MMSE) reveals that he is not disorientated but does show mild short-term memory loss. Which is the single most appropriate course of action? ★ ★

A Advise him again verbally that he needs to inform the DVLA

B Advise him verbally of your responsibility to disclose his diagnosis to the DVLA

C Advise him verbally that he should stop driving from now on

D Disclose his diagnosis to the DVLA

E Write to him again, advising that he needs to inform the DVLA

26. A 20-year-old woman has panic attacks when she has to attend formal meetings at work. She also feels anxious when she meets her friends in the pub. Which is the single most likely diagnosis? ★ ★

A Adjustment disorder

B Generalized anxiety disorder

C Panic disorder

D Post-traumatic stress disorder

E Social phobia

27. A 60-year-old man asks for a repeat prescription for diazepam. He says that his general practitioner (GP) started him on this treatment 3 months ago when he was anxious and depressed after losing his job. Which is the single most appropriate course of action? ★ ★

A Call his usual GP to arrange an appointment for him in 1 week's time

B Change his prescription to an antidepressant drug, and explain that this would be a more appropriate treatment

C Explain that you cannot re-prescribe diazepam because of the risk of him becoming dependent

D Explain the risk of becoming dependent on diazepam, and then re-prescribe diazepam at half the dose for 4 more weeks

E Explain the risk of becoming dependent on diazepam, and then re-prescribe diazepam in a weekly decreasing dose

28. A 33-year-old woman with bipolar disorder is due to be started on a mood stabilizer. She has some questions about lithium. Which single symptom or sign is a common side-effect of lithium at therapeutic levels? ★ ★

A Coarse tremor

B Dysarthria

C Improvement of pre-existing skin conditions

D Thirst

E Weight loss

29. A 24-year-old man is found acting strangely in the park. He believes that MI5 are behind a plot to harm him and are keeping him under surveillance. He hears himself being commented on by a voice 'reading the news' and thinks that his thoughts are being controlled by devices on buses. Which single symptom is one of Schneider's first-rank symptoms of schizophrenia? ★ ★

A Catatonia

B Ideas of reference

C Persecutory delusions

D Poverty of speech

E Third-person auditory hallucinations

30. A 26-year-old woman has emotional lability and a mildly depressed mood. She feels 'numb' and 'empty', and has recently often acted impulsively (e.g. by shoplifting). She uses recreational drugs regularly. She has no regular partner and is unemployed. She cuts herself in response to distressing feelings but is not suicidal. Which is the single most likely diagnosis? ★ ★

A Antisocial personality disorder

B Avoidant personality disorder

C Emotionally unstable personality disorder

D Histrionic personality disorder

E Mild depressive episode

31. A 79-year-old man has personality change and worsening orientation. He has a tremor, extensor plantar reflexes, and bilateral small pupils that do not constrict in response to light but do constrict on accommodation. Which is the single most useful diagnostic investigation? ★

A Chest X-ray

B Computed tomography (CT) scan of the brain

C Electroencephalogram (EEG)

D Magnetic resonance imaging (MRI) of the brain

E Venereal Disease Research Laboratory (VDRL) test

32. The police bring a 23-year-old man to the Emergency Department, who they have detained because he was standing in the middle of the road shouting at the traffic and threatening to stab drivers. The doctor is asked to take a history and examine the patient. Which is the single most appropriate initial action for the doctor to take? ★

A Arrange for the interview to take place in a quiet, private room

B Ask the police to be present during the interview

C Remove from the room any sharp items that could be used as weapons

D Talk to the police about the patient's presentation and behaviour

E Tell another member of staff to note down where the interview will take place

33. The wife of a patient is in a distressed state. She tells her general practitioner (GP) that her husband is wandering around the house at night and that she is afraid to sleep in case he accidentally harms himself. She says that he has already drawn up a Personal Welfare Lasting Power of Attorney (LPA), which is registered at the Office of the Public Guardian, and that he has appointed her as his 'attorney' to make decisions on his behalf. The GP knows that the patient has a diagnosis of dementia, although it is 6 months since he last saw him. The patient's wife asks the GP to prescribe some sedative medication, adding that her husband is quite happy to take a tablet at night. Which is the single most appropriate response for the GP to make? ★★★

A Advise the patient's wife that he would need to talk to other members of the family as well before he prescribed any medication

B Explain to the patient's wife that an LPA does not cover decisions about medical treatment

C Explain to the patient's wife that he would need to see her husband to assess whether he lacks the capacity to decide whether or not to take sedative medication

D Explain to the patient's wife that she cannot give consent on behalf of her husband for him to prescribe medication

E Prescribe a small dose of sedative medication for the patient and see him in 1 week

34. A 23-year-old woman has had psychological and somatic symptoms of anxiety for 3 weeks, which mostly occur when she has to drive her car in the city. This is the first time she has suffered from these symptoms. Which is the single most appropriate treatment? ★★★★

A Anxiety management training

B Behavioural therapy

C Brief psychodynamic psychotherapy

D A selective serotonin reuptake inhibitor (SSRI)

E A tricyclic antidepressant

35. A 3-year-old boy has been referred to the paediatrician and child psychiatrist for assessment. He was late in starting to talk and is falling behind his peers at nursery. He is thought to have mild learning disability. His parents have some questions. Which single statement about mild learning disability is appropriate when counselling the parents? ★ ★ ★ ★

A A specific cause cannot be identified in 50% of cases

B Epilepsy occurs in 70% of people with mild learning disability

C Fragile X syndrome is an X-linked recessive condition that can cause mild learning disability

D Only a very small number of people with mild learning disability are capable of working in adulthood

E The expected intelligence quotient (IQ) range is between 20 and 35

36. A 6-year-old boy does not talk and will not play with other children. He is only interested in toy cars and lines them up in a particular order. His teacher says that he cannot read or write like the other children, and that he has temper tantrums for no obvious reason. Which is the single most likely diagnosis? ★ ★ ★ ★

A Asperger's syndrome

B Autism

C Normal child

D Obsessive–compulsive disorder

E Rett's syndrome

37. A 30-year-old man with paranoid schizophrenia has not responded to two consecutive 8-week trials of olanzapine and risperidone at therapeutic doses. Which is the single most appropriate course of action? ★ ★ ★ ★

A Combine olanzapine and risperidone

B Commence clozapine

C Commence haloperidol

D Commence risperidone long-acting injection

E Continue olanzapine at a higher dose

38. A 35-year-old man was prescribed an antidepressant 8 months ago for a moderately severe depressive episode. This was his first depressive episode. He now feels that he has almost recovered and wants to know when he can stop taking the antidepressant. Which is the single most appropriate piece of advice? ★ ★ ★ ★

A He must take the tablets for the rest of his life

B He should continue the medication for 1 to 2 months after he has recovered

C He should continue the medication for 4 to 6 months after he has recovered

D He should continue the medication for 1 year after he has recovered

E He should stop the antidepressants immediately if he feels that he is back to normal

39. A 30-year-old man with paranoid schizophrenia on the ward becomes very agitated one night. He is pacing around, talking to himself, and appears to be responding to hallucinations. He is verbally aggressive and hostile to staff and other patients. He has a history of violence when unwell. Simple de-escalation techniques have failed to calm the situation, but he is willing to take medication. Which is the single most appropriate management? ★ ★ ★ ★

A Give clozapine 50 mg orally and review in 1 hour

B Give haloperidol 10 mg intramuscularly (IM) and review in 1 hour

C Give lorazepam 2 mg orally and review in 1 hour

D Give olanzapine 20 mg IM and review in 1 hour

E Request police presence on the ward

40. A 31-year-old single mother discloses that she regularly cuts herself in front of her 6-year-old son and that he often becomes distressed if he thinks she is feeling sad. She is not taking him to school every day. Which is the single most appropriate course of action? ★ ★ ★ ★

A Contact the school to find out whether her son's teacher has any concerns about him

B Find out whether she has any extra support, such as a family member, to help look after her son

C Refer to the police and social services immediately

D Speak to a senior colleague and the designated child protection lead

E Tell her that if she does not stop self-harming, you will have to take action

41. A 22-year-old woman has recurrent depressive episodes. Her main symptoms are low mood, anhedonia, insomnia, and weight loss secondary to poor appetite. She has had adverse reactions to selective serotonin reuptake inhibitors (SSRIs) in the past. Which would be the single most appropriate medication to prescribe? ★ ★ ★ ★

A Citalopram

B Fluoxetine

C Mirtazapine

D Paroxetine

E Sertraline

42. A 47-year-old man with paranoid schizophrenia has been known to his mental health team for 15 years. He has needed eight admissions during that time. He has recently deteriorated due to non-compliance with medication and is threatening his neighbours with violence. He is now in a very similar state to that with which he has presented in the past when unwell. He is refusing to agree to admission to hospital for treatment. Which is the single most appropriate section of the Mental Health Act 2007 (England and Wales) to use? ★ ★ ★ ★

A Section 2

B Section 3

C Section 5

D Section 17

E Section 136

43. A 48-year-old woman is admitted to hospital for routine surgery. She takes once-daily lithium for treatment of bipolar disorder. Which is the single correct time to take her blood to check plasma levels of lithium? ★ ★ ★ ★

A Immediately before her dose

B 2 hours after her dose

C 8 hours after her dose

D 12 hours after her dose

E 20 hours after her dose

44. A 35-year-old man who is opiate-dependent is considering tackling his addiction. In discussing treatment options, which is the single most appropriate piece of advice to include? ★ ★ ★ ★

A Methadone has a shorter half-life than heroin

B Naltrexone is an opiate agonist and is an alternative to methadone

C Opiate withdrawal results in death if untreated

D Opiate withdrawal causes restlessness, abdominal pain, and anxiety

E The withdrawal syndrome will begin 2 to 3 days after heroin was last taken

45. A previously healthy 78-year-old man has a severe depressive illness. He has not responded to various treatments so far, and his consultant wants to prescribe a tricyclic antidepressant. Which is the single most important investigation before commencing treatment? ★ ★ ★ ★

A Computed tomography (CT) scan of the brain

B Electrocardiogram (ECG)

C Full blood count

D Urea and electrolytes

E Urinalysis

ANSWERS

1. B ★   OHCS 10th edn → pp. 364, 376

Alcohol withdrawal can cause delirium tremens, which is characterized by florid visual or tactile hallucinations, typically of small creatures. This is relatively common in drinkers who are suddenly admitted to hospital, and a detailed alcohol history should always be taken to try to prevent withdrawal using appropriate medication.

→ http://www.nice.org.uk/guidance/CG115

2. D ★   OHCS 10th edn → p. 192

All patients who have a delayed presentation (more than 8 hours) after paracetamol overdose should have *N*-acetylcysteine started immediately.

3. E ★

In Munchausen syndrome, or factitious illness, affected individuals fake illness in order to gain medical attention. Often, reasonably serious symptoms, such as blood in the stools or urine, can be falsified. These cannot be reproduced when the person is being directly observed. Malingering is the term used for people who feign illness for another gain (e.g. financial benefit or avoidance of work). Hypochondriasis refers to an excessive worry about illness, and these patients may often have vague medical symptoms such as palpitations or abdominal pain.

4. C ★

These are the classic signs of acute opioid intoxication.

5. A ★

The key here is that the person is excessively concerned with an imagined abnormality in his physical appearance, which is affecting his life. It is not an obsession and is not affecting the mood. The social withdrawal is occurring because of the concern about the feature, rather than because of anxiety. Hypochondriasis is a fear of serious illness, rather than concern about physical features.

6. D ★   OHCS 10th edn → p. 376

It is not the amount drunk, or the quality of what a person drinks, but the effect that it has on their life that characterizes dependence.

7. E ★   OHCS 10th edn → p. 340

Olanzapine is a commonly used atypical antipsychotic drug. These have different side-effects from typical antipsychotic drugs such as haloperidol and chlorpromazine. Lorazepam is a benzodiazepine. Mirtazapine is an antidepressant.

8. C ★   OHCS 10th edn → p. 344

Depression following an MI is associated with a poor prognosis, although the evidence that treatment of depression improves this is equivocal. Tricyclic antidepressants increase the risk of MI, so they should not be used in patients with ischaemic heart disease. SSRIs may have a protective effect. Benzodiazepines do not treat depression. MAOIs are used only rarely for depression nowadays, due to their potentially lethal interactions.

→ Anon. Depression, antidepressants and heart disease. *Drug Ther Bull.* 2008;**46**:29–32.

9. D ★

Hypothyroidism is a recognized cause of depression, and it also causes physical symptoms, including lethargy, weight gain, constipation, dry skin and hair, and oedema. Recognition of these symptoms should point towards investigation of thyroid function to guide appropriate treatment.

10. C ★   OHCS 10th edn → p. 350

Although some of these symptoms may occur in any of the options given, the young age, combination of symptoms, and complete resolution within a short time make a panic attack the most likely diagnosis.

11. B ★   OHCS 10th edn → p. 404

Although this woman has signed a consent form, a patient can withdraw consent at any time. Although she has a history of obsessive–compulsive disorder, which would satisfy the definition of a mental disorder under the Mental Health Act 2007 (England and Wales) or the Mental Health (Care and Treatment) (Scotland) Act 2003, she cannot be detained under the Act to allow medical or surgical treatment to continue. The fact that she has pre-eclampsia does not constitute a danger to herself or others (i.e. her babies) under the Act, as this risk is not arising from her mental disorder.

12. A ★   OHCS 10th edn → p. 360

→ http://research.bmh.manchester.ac.uk/cmhs/research/centrefor-suicideprevention/nci (key findings (suicide) from the National Confidential Inquiry into Suicide and Homicide by People with a Mental Illness)

13. C ★   OHCS 10th edn → p. 376

A raised MCV and GGT are indicative of problem drinking. Two or more positive responses are needed on the CAGE questionnaire. Urate levels are raised in about 50% of all people with drinking problems, but they are only useful as screening tests for men, as they are poor discriminators in women. The AUDIT is a simple 10-question test developed by the World Health Organization (WHO) to determine whether a person's alcohol consumption may be harmful. The test was designed to be used internationally and was validated in a study using patients from six countries. Questions 1 to 3 deal with alcohol consumption, Questions 4 to 6 relate to alcohol dependence, and Questions 7 to 10 consider alcohol-related problems.

→ http://apps.who.int/iris/bitstream/10665/67205/1/WHO_MSD_ MSB_01.6a.pdf

14. **A** ★

Cocaine abuse has sympathomimetic effects and causes tachycardia, hypertension, and pupillary dilatation. Heroin has the opposite effect. Solvent abuse causes signs similar to those of alcohol intoxication but may also include hallucinations. Psilocybin, which is found in 'magic mushrooms', also causes hallucinations. Oxazepam is a benzodiazepine.

15. **C** ★

In delirium and a post-ictal state, there would be alteration in the level of consciousness. In Alzheimer's disease, the person would have generalized cognitive impairment that is progressive. Normal-pressure hydrocephalus usually presents with a triad of ataxia, dementia, and urinary incontinence.

16. **C** ★   OHCS 10th edn → p. 409

The Mental Capacity Act 2005 (England and Wales) provides a statutory framework to empower and protect vulnerable people who are not able to make their own decisions. It is underpinned by five key principles:

1. Every adult is presumed to have capacity unless it is proven otherwise.
2. Individuals must be supported to make their own decisions.
3. Individuals retain the right to make what might be viewed as unwise or eccentric decisions.
4. Any action taken on behalf of individuals who lack capacity must be done in their best interests.
5. Any action taken on behalf of people who lack capacity must be the least restrictive option.

In this case, the patient has capacity and is not suffering from any mental impairment (e.g. psychotic depression or dementia). Therefore, although it seems an unwise decision, she has the right to refuse surgery. However, in complicated and life-threatening cases such as this, it is always wise to seek a second opinion and, if necessary, to involve your Trust's legal department. Note that Scotland has a separate legal framework—the Adults with Incapacity (Scotland) Act 2000.

→ http://www.gov.uk/government/publications/mental-capacity-act-code-of-practice

→ http://www.gov.scot/Publications/2003/03/16933/21228

17. C ★   OHCS 10th edn → p. 352

An obsession is a stereotyped, purposeless word, idea, or phrase that comes into the mind and that originates from the person, rather than from outside. The patient realizes that it is not true.

18. C ★

Bradypnoea, bradycardia, and pinpoint pupils strongly suggest opioid overdose. The treatment for this is intramuscular and intravenous naloxone.

19. E ★   OHCS 10th edn → p. 366

The history of strokes, together with the progressive dementia, points to vascular dementia caused by multiple infarcts. Alzheimer's disease is a possibility, but the vascular history suggests otherwise. Lewy body dementia is characterized by hallucinations, visuo-perceptual defects, and a fluctuating course. Fronto-temporal dementia, or Pick's disease, is characterized by frontal lobe signs such as disinhibition.

20. A ★   OHCS 10th edn → p. 344

In mild depression, watchful waiting and review is the first-line strategy. Although this woman has low mood and lack of energy, she is functioning at work and socially, and has no physical symptoms and no suicidal ideation.

→ http://www.nice.org.uk/guidance/CG90

21. B ★   OHCS 10th edn → p. 350

All of these approaches could be used, but as anxiety disorders are maintained by fears about the nature and consequences of symptoms, an explanation of the condition is the first step in treatment. Anxious patients do not concentrate well, especially when given new information. Therefore, writing down the key points so that the patient can read them at home is the optimum approach.

22. E ★

Chronic alcohol consumption can result in thiamine deficiency due to inadequate nutritional intake, impaired uptake in the bowel, and impaired metabolism. Thiamine deficiency can lead to alcohol-induced brain damage, so thiamine should be replaced intravenously if patients with alcohol abuse show signs of possible brain damage. The other medications have roles in treating various addictions but are not appropriate in this case.

23. D ★   OHCS 10th edn → p. 346

All of the other side-effect profiles are prominent in patients who are prescribed tricyclic antidepressants. Confusion is more likely to occur in elderly patients who are prescribed tricyclic antidepressants, and this, together with signs such as dry mouth, is due to the anticholinergic effects of these drugs. Their adrenergic antagonism may cause cardiovascular effects. Citalopram is a selective serotonin reuptake inhibitor (SSRI).

24. B ★   OHCS 10th edn → p. 340

Risperidone is an atypical antipsychotic and is associated with hyperprolactinaemia. This may result in gynaecomastia and galactorrhoea in men, and disturbance of the menstrual cycle in women. The side-effects of risperidone sometimes include sexual dysfunction and weight gain.

25. E ★★

The General Medical Council (GMC) has clearly stated that, for several conditions (including dementia), doctors should not only advise patients of the possibility of having to stop driving, but should also take steps to ensure that the relevant statutory authorities are informed of breaches of regulation if there is reasonable concern about public safety. Initially this should be done by informing the patient of the need to let the DVLA know about their condition. The fact that this patient is not disorientated, his short-term memory loss is mild, and he was only diagnosed a year ago would suggest that you do not have to make an immediate clinical decision that he is unfit to continue driving until the DVLA has assessed him.

→ Breen DA, Breen DP, Moore JW, Breen PA, O'Neill D. Driving and dementia. BMJ. 2007;**334**:1365–9.

→ http://www.gmc-uk.org/guidance/ethical_guidance/confidentiality.asp

→ http://www.gov.uk/browse/driving/disability-health-condition

26. E ★★   OHCS 10th edn → p. 350

There are many different types of anxiety disorder. The fact that all of the patient's symptoms occur in social situations makes social phobia the most likely diagnosis.

27. E ★★   OHCS 10th edn → p. 356

Long-term use of benzodiazepines runs the risk of creating dependency. However, suddenly stopping them may cause a withdrawal syndrome. If this man has run out of diazepam, there is a risk that he will develop withdrawal syndrome if he has to wait a week to see his usual GP. Antidepressants will not help the withdrawal. A reducing regime can be used to wean him off the diazepam, but this should be supervised.

28. D ★★   OHCS 10th edn → pp. 348–9

Lithium has a narrow therapeutic index, which means that the difference between effective and toxic doses is small. Thirst is a common side-effect. Fine tremor is also common, and weight gain and skin rash can occur. At toxic levels, dysarthria can occur.

29. **E** ★ ★   OHCS 10th edn → p. 336

Schneider's first-rank symptoms of schizophrenia are symptoms that, if present, are strongly suggestive of schizophrenia. They include the following:[*]

- auditory hallucinations: hearing thoughts spoken aloud, hearing voices referring to oneself in the third person, auditory hallucinations in the form of a commentary
- thought withdrawal, insertion, and interruption
- thought broadcasting
- somatic hallucinations
- delusional perception
- feelings or actions experienced as being generated or influenced by external agents.

30. **C** ★ ★   OHCS 10th edn → p. 380

There are a number of personality disorders, each of which has its own unique features. They all start in childhood or late adolescence and are patterns of inner experience and behaviour that remain stable throughout life and are different from that which would normally be expected in the society in which the person lives. There are two types of emotionally unstable personality disorder—borderline and impulsive. In the borderline type, the person tends to form intense relationships and have rapid fluctuations in mood, with impulsivity, disturbed self-image, recurrent self-harm, and chronic feelings of emptiness.

31. **E** ★

Neurosyphilis is an uncommon cause of psychiatric illness but is suggested by the Argyll Robertson pupils, as described in the question. These are a highly specific sign of neurosyphilis.

32. **D** ★

Careful consideration has to be given to team safety when assessing potentially dangerous patients. The police may know the patient and be able to provide valuable information such as a history of mental health problems or drug use. In addition, the information that the doctor is given by the police may well influence how and where the patient is seen. For example, it may become clear that the doctor needs to be accompanied by another health-care professional. The police may well have to leave, and their information should be sought early. Although a quiet, private room may help to calm the patient, it may put the doctor in a dangerous situation. Any room that is used should have all potentially dangerous objects removed from it, and the doctor should always place him- or herself between the door and the patient. Although having the

---

[*] Source data from Schneider K, *Clinical Psychopathology*, New York: Grune & Stratton, 1959.

police present for the interview may seem a sensible option, it will compromise confidentiality, and if the patient has paranoid thoughts or beliefs, a police presence may well exacerbate these. It is better to ask a member of the health-care staff whether there is a need for the doctor to be accompanied.

33. C ★★★   OHCS 10th edn → p. 409

Under the Mental Capacity Act 2005 (England and Wales), a Personal Welfare LPA does not come into effect until the patient has lost capacity to consent, even though it may be registered with the Office of the Public Guardian. As the GP has not seen the patient for 6 months, he does not know whether he has capacity to decide for himself whether to take medication. Although he has a diagnosis of dementia, which may have affected his capacity under the Act, every adult has the right to make their own decisions and must be assumed to have capacity to make them, unless it is proved otherwise. Until the GP has assessed the patient, he cannot assume that he does not have capacity. If the GP has assessed the patient and has judged that he does lack capacity to decide whether to take this medication, and that prescribing such medication is in his best interests, then the Personal Welfare LPA would allow his wife to give or refuse consent to the administration of treatment by a person providing health-care. Note that a separate Act—the Adults with Incapacity (Scotland) Act 2000—is in place in Scotland.

→ http://www.gov.uk/government/publications/mental-capacity-act-code-of-practice

→ http://www.gov.scot/Publications/2003/03/16933/21228

34. A ★★★★   OHCS 10th edn → p. 350

Anxiety management training is a form of cognitive behavioural therapy that has the best record for the treatment of anxiety. Behavioural therapy with graded exposure to anxiety-provoking stimuli may be useful in some specific cases. Paroxetine (an SSRI) can help to treat social anxiety, but non-pharmacological measures should be tried first.

35. A ★★★★   OHCS 10th edn → p. 216

More often than not, a cause cannot be identified, although genetic causes should be considered, as they may have implications for genetic counselling. Fragile X syndrome is not X-linked recessive but is caused by an expansion of triplet repeats on the X chromosome through successive generations. Epilepsy can occur in learning disability, but only in about 30% of individuals. There is a spectrum of learning disability, and many adults will be able to be supported in finding suitable employment. In mild learning disability, the expected IQ is approximately 50–70; in moderate learning disability, it is 35–50, and in severe learning disability, it is 20–35. However, the IQ provides no information about individual strengths and weaknesses, so it is not the best way of classifying learning disability.

36. B ★★★★   OHCS 10th edn → p. 372

These are all features that suggest a diagnosis on the autistic spectrum. Autism is a pervasive developmental disorder with features that include the following:

- impaired communication: in the most severe cases, there is no language at all, no imaginative play, and echolalia (repeating other people's words)
- impaired social interaction (e.g. not responding to other people's emotions)
- restricted, repetitive, and stereotyped patterns of movement, behaviours, and interests (e.g. liking rigid routines and becoming upset when these do not occur, enjoying activities such as lining toys up or spinning wheels repeatedly)
- onset before the age of 3 years.

Asperger's syndrome is classified by some as being at one end of the spectrum. However, language is retained in Asperger's syndrome, although it is qualitatively different. Rett's syndrome occurs in girls.

37. B ★★★★   OHCS 10th edn → p. 340

In England and Wales, there are published guidelines on the use of clozapine in the treatment of resistant schizophrenia.

→ http://www.nice.org.uk/guidance/CG82

38. C ★★★★

If antidepressants are stopped too soon, about 50% of patients will relapse. Antidepressants should be withdrawn over a period of several weeks.

→ http://www.nice.org.uk/guidance/CG90

39. C ★★★★   OHCS 10th edn → p. 363

You should familiarize yourself with your local Trust's rapid tranquillization policy for cases such as this. In general, start with simple de-escalation techniques (talking calmly, using non-hostile body language, etc.), and, if necessary, offer oral medication first, only moving on to intramuscular administration if the patient refuses oral treatment. A benzodiazepine such as lorazepam is a good starting point, and you should review the situation regularly. If this is not effective, an antipsychotic should be prescribed. First-generation antipsychotics such as haloperidol are no longer the first-line approach, because of the risk of dystonic side-effects. Olanzapine would be an appropriate choice, but note that it cannot be given within 1 hour of lorazepam.

40. D ★★★★

In the interest of safeguarding children, concerns like this should not be ignored. According to recommendations from *Good Medical Practice*, all doctors have a duty to consider the interests of children who may be in the care of adult patients. There are local systems in place to discuss non-urgent concerns, and all Trusts will have a designated lead for child protection.

→ http://www.gmc-uk.org/guidance/ethical_guidance/13257.asp

41. C ★★★★ OHCS 10th edn → p. 341

Fluoxetine, paroxetine, sertraline, and citalopram are all SSRIs. For patients who cannot tolerate SSRIs, the next choice would be mirtazapine, which is a reuptake inhibitor and receptor blocker that affects the levels of noradrenaline (norepinephrine) and serotonin in the synapses.

→ http://www.nice.org.uk/guidance/CG90

42. B ★★★★ OHCS 10th edn → p. 408

The Mental Health Act 2007 applies to England and Wales. Scotland has a separate Act—the Mental Health (Care and Treatment) (Scotland) Act 2003.

- Section 2 is a (maximum) 28-day section for assessment of a patient with a mental disorder. It is used if the diagnosis is not clear.
- Section 3 is a (maximum) 6-month section for treatment. It is only used if the patient is well known to the health-care professionals and the symptoms are consistent with the type that they suffer from when unwell.
- Section 5 is an emergency holding power, used by nurses (Section 5(4)) or doctors (Section 5(2)) to detain an informal patient who is already an inpatient.
- Section 17 is the part of the Mental Health Act that allows the Responsible Clinician to grant a detained inpatient leave from the hospital.
- Section 136 is an emergency section used by the police to bring a person in a public place whom they suspect is suffering from a mental disorder to a place of safety in order that they may be assessed.

→ http://www.legislation.gov.uk/ukpga/2007/12/contents

→ http://www.gov.scot/Publications/2008/09/24090333/1

43. D ★★★★ OHCS 10th edn → p. 348

Drug levels may need to be checked for a number of drugs which have a narrow dose range—a small window in which the drug is effective, but not toxic. To be effective, peak levels should be within the therapeutic range, but not be so high as to cause toxic side-effects, and trough levels should stay within therapeutic range. The metabolism of a drug can be affected by a number of factors, e.g. the person's metabolism, their physical health, other drugs that they take, etc. Trough levels are checked just before a dose. Peak levels are checked at some point soon after a dose. Study of different drugs has determined when levels should be checked for different dosing regimes, and most organizations will have protocols for the testing of common drug levels, guided by the *British National Formulary* (*BNF*). Lithium is a commonly used psychiatric drug that requires monitoring, especially at a time of change in the patient's circumstances.

→ http://www.bnf.org (registration required)

44. D ★★★★   OHCS 10th edn → p. 374

Opiate withdrawal is an unpleasant experience but does not result in death in healthy individuals. Symptoms include restlessness, anxiety, insomnia, abdominal pain, nausea, diarrhoea, yawning, and piloerection. Methadone is a long-acting opiate, with a long half-life, which is taken orally once a day and so reduces the 'rush' that is caused by injecting heroin. Naltrexone is an opiate antagonist that can be used after completing detoxification, to reduce the risk of relapse.

45. B ★★★★

Tricyclic antidepressants can slow cardiac conduction and may cause arrhythmias and heart block. This is particularly dangerous in the elderly, in whom the side-effect of postural hypotension may also be a problem.

Ophthalmology

Venki Sundaram

Ophthalmology principally aims to prevent visual loss, restore visual function, and relieve ocular discomfort. The majority of the pathology can be directly visualized and thus requires proficient ocular examination techniques and visual recognition skills.

Another distinguishing aspect of ophthalmology is the overlap between medical and surgical conditions. Common systemic diseases such as diabetes and hypertension have ocular features, and diseases involving every organ of the body can have ocular manifestations. A thorough medical knowledge is paramount, as is the ability to collaborate with other medical teams. Intraocular surgery for conditions such as cataract is technically challenging, as ocular tissues are so delicate. It therefore requires high levels of fine hand–eye coordination.

As an ophthalmologist, you will be faced both with acute eye conditions, some of which are sight-threatening and require prompt diagnosis and management, and with chronic conditions, which require monitoring and treatment for many years. You will be exposed to patients of all ages, from premature babies to the elderly, so good communication with a wide range of patient groups and their families is essential. Patients often say that what they fear most is losing their sight. Therefore, empathy and support for patients with debilitating visual impairment are imperative.

The questions in this chapter will test your knowledge of acute emergency ophthalmic presentations and the understanding and interpretation of ophthalmic examination, as well as ocular conditions that have systemic associations. In addition, questions relating to ophthalmic risk factors, communication, and probity are included. Eye problems can be daunting to many medical students and doctors. Through practice in examining patients and recognizing key conditions, confidence can be gained in how best to manage these patients and, importantly, when to refer them to other specialties. Ophthalmology incorporates a unique and appealing mix of medical and surgical conditions. It is a rapidly advancing specialty with recent significant advances in diagnostic and therapeutic options. It also provides an opportunity for a good work–life balance.

QUESTIONS

1. A 72-year-old man has painless, sudden of loss of vision in his right eye. Twenty-four hours later, visual acuity in his right eye is limited to counting fingers, and there is a carotid bruit on the right side. His blood pressure (BP) is 155/100 mmHg. His fundus appearance is shown in Figure 5.1 (see Colour Plate section). Which is the single most likely diagnosis? ★

A Central retinal artery occlusion

B Central retinal vein occlusion

C Papilloedema

D Rhegmatogenous retinal detachment

E Transient ischaemic attack

2. A 69-year-old woman with hypermetropia has had increasing left ocular pain, redness, and blurring of vision for 6 hours. She is seeing haloes around bright lights, and she feels nauseated. Her left eye is shown in Figure 5.2 (see Colour Plate section). Which is the single most likely diagnosis? ★

A Acute angle closure

B Anterior scleritis

C Bacterial conjunctivitis

D Iritis

E Subconjunctival haemorrhage

3. A 72-year-old woman has sudden loss of vision in her right eye. She has been experiencing temporal headache, jaw ache, and shoulder pain for the last 2 weeks. Her visual acuity in the right eye is limited to seeing hand movements. The appearance of her fundus is shown in Figure 5.3 (see Colour Plate section). Which single investigation would be most likely to support the diagnosis? ★

A Blood cultures

B Computed tomography (CT) scan of the head

C Erythrocyte sedimentation rate (ESR)

D Fluorescein angiography

E Full blood count

4. A 54-year-old woman has had increasing severe right ocular pain for 3 days, which is now affecting her sleep. Her vision is unaffected, but she has considerable ocular tenderness. Her right eye is shown in Figure 5.4 (see Colour Plate section). Which single systemic condition is most commonly associated with her ocular condition? ★

A Acute lymphocytic leukaemia

B Bacterial endocarditis

C Malignant carcinoma of the colon

D Multiple sclerosis

E Rheumatoid arthritis

5. A 6-year-old boy has had increasing fever, malaise, and right lid swelling over the last 48 hours. His eyelid is shown in Figure 5.5 (see Colour Plate section). When the eyelid is opened with difficulty, he has conjunctival chemosis and mild proptosis, with limitation of upgaze. His temperature is 38.6°C. Which is the single most appropriate treatment? ★

A Intravenous broad-spectrum antibiotics

B Oral antihistamines

C Oral broad-spectrum antibiotics

D Systemic steroids

E Topical antibiotics

6. A 22-year-old man is hit in his right eye with a glass bottle. His vision is 6/24 unaided, and his eye is shown in Figure 5.6 (see Colour Plate section). Which is the single most serious complication of this injury? ★

A Cataract

B Endophthalmitis

C Hyphaema

D Iridodialysis

E Lens subluxation

7. A 27-year-old woman has accidentally splashed an alkaline detergent in both eyes. She is in considerable discomfort and has marked diffuse bilateral conjunctival injection and hazy corneas. Which is the single most appropriate immediate management? ★

A Application of eye pads

B Irrigation with normal saline

C Limbal stem cell transplant

D Topical antibiotic

E Topical vitamin C

8. A 33-year-old man has had increasing diplopia, drooping of the left upper lid, and headache over the last 2 days. There is a complete left ptosis and the left pupil is dilated. The left eye is depressed and abducted, and eye movements are limited in all directions, except downgaze and abduction. Which single condition must be investigated for immediately? ★

A Aponeurotic ptosis

B Myasthenia gravis

C Orbital myositis

D Posterior communicating artery aneurysm

E Thyroid eye disease

9. A 77-year-old woman had uneventful right cataract surgery 3 days ago. She now has increasing pain, redness, and reduced vision in this eye. Her vision is 6/60, and there is marked conjunctival injection and anterior chamber inflammation with a 1-mm hypopyon. The fundal view is hazy. Which is the single most likely diagnosis? ★

A Acute angle-closure glaucoma

B Bacterial conjunctivitis

C Bacterial endophthalmitis

D Iritis

E Scleritis

10. A 45-year-old woman complains of irritable eyes and double vision when she looks to her side. She is concerned that her facial appearance has changed in recent months and that she has had some weight loss despite an increased appetite. There is moderate conjunctival vessel injection, and the sclera is visible between her upper lids and cornea. There is proptosis of both eyes. On extreme lateral gaze, there is limitation of eye movement and diplopia. Which is the single most likely cause of her eye problems? ★

A Carotid–cavernous fistula

B Optic nerve glioma

C Orbital haemangioma

D Orbital myositis

E Thyroid eye disease

11. A 66-year-old man who smokes 15 cigarettes a day has unequal pupil size. His visual acuity is unaffected and his right pupil is smaller, becoming more apparent in darker conditions. His pupils react normally to light and there is mild right upper lid ptosis. Which is the single most appropriate test to confirm the diagnosis of his pupil abnormality? ★★

A Chest X-ray

B Erythrocyte sedimentation rate (ESR)

C Magnetic resonance imaging (MRI) scan of the head

D Topical cocaine eye drops

E Topical phenylephrine eye drops

12. A 47-year-old man is referred after being found on annual check-up by his optician to have raised intraocular pressures. He has type 2 diabetes and his uncle receives treatment for glaucoma. His visual acuity is 6/6 in both eyes, with glasses for myopia, and his intraocular pressures are 34 mmHg in the right eye and 36 mmHg in the left eye. Which single risk factor is most important for the development of glaucoma? ★★

A Age

B Diabetes

C Family history of glaucoma

D Myopia

E Raised intraocular pressure level

13. A 41-year-old woman has had gradual visual loss in her left eye over the last few years. Her optician initially commented that she had an early cataract that was too 'immature' for surgery to be considered, but this has now progressed. Her visual acuity is 6/60 in the left eye and 6/6 in the right eye. There is a mild left cortical cataract, and fundal examination reveals a total rhegmatogenous retinal detachment. Which is the single most appropriate course of action? ★★

A Explain in detail the pathological processes involved in developing a retinal detachment

B Explain that she has developed a retinal detachment, and discuss the surgical options for reattaching the retina and the likely visual prognosis

C Explore why she did not suspect that something more serious was causing her visual loss

D Recommend that she pursues legal action against her optician for delay in diagnosis of a retinal detachment

E Tell her that she has a retinal detachment and is likely to go blind in the left eye, but that she still has the sight in her other eye

14. A 68-year-old woman with hypertension has had gradually decreasing vision in her left eye. Her visual acuity is 6/36, improving to 6/9 with pinhole testing, in this eye. Which is the single most likely diagnosis? ★ ★ ★

A Cataract

B Central retinal artery occlusion

C Central retinal vein occlusion

D Dry age-related degeneration

E Glaucoma

15. A 58-year-old man with hypertension who has previously undergone a renal transplant complains of floaters and blurring of vision in his right eye. He is highly myopic, and his visual acuity is 6/18. Fundoscopy shows peripheral areas of yellow-white retina, surrounded by haemorrhage. Which is the single most likely diagnosis? ★ ★ ★

A Central retinal vein occlusion

B Choroidal melanoma

C Cytomegalovirus retinitis

D Hypertensive retinopathy

E Retinal detachment

16. A 65-year-old woman with multiple sclerosis has reduced right visual acuity. She has type 2 diabetes and underwent squint surgery to her right eye as a child. Her right visual acuity is 6/36 with glasses, and there is no pinhole improvement. A swinging flashlight test shows a right relative afferent pupillary defect. Which is the single most likely diagnosis? ★ ★ ★ ★

A Amblyopia

B Background diabetic retinopathy

C Cataract

D Diabetic macular oedema

E Optic neuritis

17. A 73-year-old man had routine right cataract surgery 2 weeks ago. At his post-operative visit, it was found that his vision is not as clear as he was expecting. Refraction and review of the operation notes reveal a significant (4 dioptre) refractive error due to an intraocular lens of the wrong power being inserted during surgery. Which is the single most appropriate course of action? ★ ★ ★ ★

A Advise the patient that things will settle and that it can take time for the brain to adjust to the new vision

B Apologize and explain that an error has occurred, and involve a senior colleague who can discuss the various management options

C Apologize and explain that the wrong lens was inserted during the operation because the surgeon was handed a lens of the wrong power

D Apologize and explain that some natural lens fragments have unfortunately been retained in the eye and that a further operation is needed to remove these and replace the lens

E Do not mention that an error has occurred, and advise the patient to visit his optician, who can 'fine-tune' his vision

ANSWERS

1. A ★   OHCS 10th edn → p. 437

A pale fundus with a 'cherry-red' spot at the macula is classically found in central retinal artery occlusions. Hypertension and sources of potential emboli (e.g. carotid artery disease) are risk factors for developing this condition.

2. A ★   OHCS 10th edn → p. 432

Ocular pain and nausea are due to the acute rise in intraocular pressure. This also causes corneal oedema, with reduced vision and glare symptoms. Examination findings are typically ciliary vessel injection, mid-dilated pupil, shallow anterior chamber depth, and high intraocular pressure (>40 mmHg). Increasing age and hypermetropia are risk factors for developing acute angle closure.

3. C ★   OHCS 10th edn → p. 436

This woman has a left anterior ischaemic optic neuropathy, secondary to giant cell arteritis (temporal arteritis). A very raised ESR is typically found, and patients can experience temporal headache, jaw pain, and myalgia. The posterior ciliary arteries may be affected by the arteritis, resulting in an anterior ischaemic optic neuropathy causing dramatic visual loss and a swollen disc with flame-shaped haemorrhages.

4. E ★   OHCS 10th edn → p. 430

This woman has a right diffuse anterior scleritis. This is associated with an underlying autoimmune condition in nearly 50% of cases, of which rheumatoid arthritis is the most common.

5. A ★   OHCS 10th edn → p. 420

This boy has a right-sided orbital cellulitis, which usually arises from bacterial spread from adjacent sinuses. This differs from preseptal cellulitis, as congestion from orbital spread results in chemosis, proptosis, and restriction of eye movement, in addition to eyelid involvement. This is an emergency, requiring urgent intravenous antibiotics and possible drainage of any sinus abscess. A delay in treatment can result in complications such as optic nerve compression and meningeal spread.

6. B ★   OHCS 10th edn → p. 742

This man has a penetrating eye injury. This requires urgent closure of the corneoscleral laceration, with appropriate antibiotic cover. A delay in management can increase the risk of developing endophthalmitis and can result in severe, permanent visual loss.

7. B ★   OHCS 10th edn → p. 742

Alkali-induced eye injuries are potentially sight-threatening, as they can cause liquefactive necrosis of ocular tissue. Immediate copious irrigation with normal saline until a neutral pH is reached can prevent further alkali penetration and destruction.

8. D ★

This man has a left-sided third nerve palsy. Pupil involvement implies a compressive cause, and the rapid, painful onset suggests an expanding lesion such as a posterior communicating artery aneurysm. This needs to be investigated immediately in order to prevent a potentially fatal sub-arachnoid haemorrhage.

9. C ★   OHCS 10th edn → p. 446

Post-operative bacterial endophthalmitis is a rare, but serious, complication of cataract surgery. Patients typically present with poor vision, pain, and significant intraocular inflammation within 2 weeks of surgery. The fundal view can be obscured by significant vitritis. Prompt recognition and management can help to prevent irreversible visual loss.

10. E ★

This woman has thyroid eye disease, which can cause ocular irritation, conjunctival vessel injection, and lid retraction. Proptosis and restriction of eye movements are secondary to enlargement of the extraocular muscles. The other conditions typically result in unilateral proptosis and are not associated with systemic symptoms.

11. D ★★   OHCS 10th edn → p. 424

This man has right-sided Horner's syndrome. This occurs because of interrupted sympathetic innervation to the eye. Topical 4% cocaine drops instilled into both eyes will only cause dilatation of the normal pupil. This is because cocaine blocks the reuptake of noradrenaline (norepinephrine) at nerve endings, causing pupil dilatation. In Horner's syndrome, no noradrenaline is secreted, so cocaine has no effect. Horner's syndrome has many causes, including Pancoast tumours of the lung.

12. E ★★   OHCS 10th edn → p. 444

Raised intraocular pressure is the strongest risk factor for the development and progression of glaucoma. Lowering of intraocular pressure is currently the only method of preventing visual field loss.

National Institute for Health and Care Excellence (2009). *Glaucoma: diagnosis and management of chronic open angle glaucoma and ocular hypertension*:

→ http://www.nice.org.uk/CG85

13. B ★★★

The news that this woman's visual loss is the result of retinal detachment, rather than cataract, is likely to come as a shock and be anxiety-provoking. Therefore, this information needs to be conveyed in a sensitive manner without placing the blame on either the patient or other professionals. Attention can then be focused on the management options available, including what possible surgery would involve and the likely visual outcome.

14. A ★★★   OHCS 10th edn → p. 442

Pinhole use focuses light entering the eye, so it can compensate for refractive errors (up to several dioptres) or conditions that cause glare such as cataract. Visual acuity improvement with pinhole testing therefore implies a refractive problem, rather than an organic problem.

15. C ★★★

Cytomegalovirus (CMV) retinitis usually only affects immunocompromised individuals. It results in areas of yellow–white retinal necrosis and haemorrhage ('pizza-pie' appearance), which can spread if not recognized and promptly treated. A raised brown fundal mass is usually evident with choroidal melanoma. Although central retinal vein occlusion can also cause retinal haemorrhage, retinal necrosis is not a feature. Significant retinal haemorrhage and retinal necrosis do not occur with retinal detachment or hypertensive retinopathy.

16. E ★★★★   OHCS 10th edn → p. 436

A relative afferent pupillary defect occurs when light shone into the affected eye causes initial dilatation of both pupils. The pupils initially dilate because the stimulus from light being shone into the affected eye is less than the stimulus of withdrawing light from the unaffected eye. This most commonly occurs in optic nerve lesions but can also be due to other gross pathology of the anterior visual pathway (e.g. total retinal detachment, optic tract lesions).

17. B ★★★★

For a variety of reasons, insertion of an intraocular lens of the wrong power during cataract surgery can unfortunately occur. Patients have a right to know about this and need to be appropriately informed of such errors and the various management options, so that they can make an informed decision on how best to rectify any visual difficulties.

The surgeon who performs the operation is ultimately responsible for the power of the intraocular lens that is inserted, even if they are handed the wrong one by a scrub nurse or assistant.

Careful preoperative selection, double-checking of all prostheses, and a safety-orientated culture in operating theatres (e.g. using the World Health Organization Safer Surgery Checklist) can reduce the risks of such errors occurring.

→ http://www.who.int/patientsafety/safesurgery/en/

Primary care

Philippa Edwards

General practitioners (GPs) are the gatekeepers of the National Health Service in the UK, and virtually all referrals to secondary care are made through them. The breadth and depth of the discipline can at times seem overwhelming, although the old adage 'common things occur commonly' still holds. GPs need to be confident in the diagnosis and management of conditions from birth to the grave, and to know their boundaries of competence and when to refer to secondary care. The complexity of the GP consultation includes the following two points:

1. Many conditions present in a relatively undifferentiated form to the GP, whose job it is to try to identify whether the condition is normal or abnormal, and whether it is serious or minor.
2. GPs develop a close professional relationship with many of their patients and may also be the point of contact for other members of the family, neighbours, and friends of the patient. This knowledge is an important aspect of their holistic approach to medicine and is much valued by their patients. As the nineteenth-century physician Sir William Osler (1849–1919) said, '*The good physician treats the disease; the great physician treats the patient who has the disease.*'

The commonest presentations to GPs in the UK are for respiratory problems, chronic disease management, musculoskeletal disorders, and psychological problems. Health promotion, in particular smoking cessation and the management of obesity, is also important in preventing chronic illness. Although many presentations are minor and self-limiting, serious illnesses also occur, and GPs need to be able to recognize them, sometimes in the early stages.

The questions in this chapter will assess your knowledge in the common areas that present, testing diagnostic skills and reasoning. They also test negotiating skills to ensure patient compliance, teamworking within the primary care setting, and risk management.

QUESTIONS

1. A 26-year-old woman has registered as a new patient, and her New Patient Health Check reveals a body mass index (BMI) of 32 kg/m². Which is the single best explanation to the patient of what the BMI means? ★

A It is a measure of cardiovascular risk

B It is a measure of how much weight a person needs to lose

C It is a representation of weight for height

D It is a way of calculating how fat the body is

E It is the ratio of hip circumference to waist circumference

2. A 44-year-old builder has acute low back pain, following heavy lifting at work the previous day. He is finding it difficult to walk. Which single feature of his presentation would warrant an urgent referral to hospital? ★

A Difficulty in passing urine

B Inability to perform a straight leg raise beyond 20°

C Pain down the back of both legs

D Reduced ankle jerks

E Use of inhaled steroids for his asthma

3. The mother of a 16-year-old girl is worried that her daughter is becoming depressed, and she knows that the girl came to see you last week. The daughter's behaviour at home has been deteriorating, and there have been a lot of arguments. The mother wants to know what the recent consultation was about and to seek your opinion about what to do. Which is the single most appropriate course of action? ★

A Advise her that she can apply to the primary care trust for access to her daughter's medical record

B Do not discuss her concerns about her daughter at all, as the daughter is over 16 years of age

C Listen to her concerns, but do not reveal information about the daughter, as the daughter has not given you consent

D Tell her a little about the recent consultation, and ask her to come back later with her daughter

E Tell her what transpired in the recent consultation, as she has a right to know as a parent

4. A 65-year-old man has had a previous small myocardial infarction. He wants advice on modifying his risk factors to prevent further health problems. Which is the single most important modifiable risk factor for stroke in this patient? ★

A Alcohol intake of 40 units per week

B Atrial fibrillation

C Body mass index of 35 kg/m²

D Previous myocardial infarction

E Raised blood pressure of 165/105 mmHg

5. A 44-year-old businessman has recently been diagnosed with high blood pressure. He does not want to take any medication. Which is the single best approach to take in the consultation to try and come to a resolution? ★

A Allow him to do what he wants to do, but tell him that he will have to see another doctor in the future

B Be friendly towards him, so that he is more likely to come back if he changes his mind

C Identify and consider his viewpoint, bringing this into the decision-making process

D Tell him all about the different medications and their side-effects, so that he has all of the information

E Tell him that he needs to take the medication which has been chosen for him or he may be at risk of harm

6. A 35-year-old woman is unable to sleep, is tired during the day, and is having problems at work as a result. Which single aspect of her history is the most likely to have a significant bearing on her presenting complaint? ★

A She drinks about 20 units of alcohol per week

B She has a 9-year-old daughter

C She has a stressful job as a teacher

D She is tearful and cannot concentrate

E She smokes ten cigarettes a day

7. A 17-year-old girl is going away to college next year. She is seeking information about the human papillomavirus (HPV) vaccine, as she missed the programme at school and is now considering having the vaccination. Which is the single most appropriate piece of information to give her about the vaccine? ★

A If she has already had sexual intercourse, she has probably already been exposed to HPV and it is not worth having the vaccination

B If she has the vaccination, it will protect her against HPV and she will not need cervical smear testing later in life

C If she suffers from eczema or asthma, she will not be able to have the vaccination because of the risk of severe allergic reactions

D The vaccination is only available as part of a primary immunization course for infants, and she is too old to be included in the 'catch-up' cohort

E The vaccination is 99% effective in preventing cervical abnormalities caused by HPV types that can lead to cervical cancer, and she is eligible to have it

8. A 52-year-old woman wants advice about mammography breast screening before her appointment. She has read a newspaper article which suggests that it may not be valuable and could even be potentially harmful. You are not aware of this evidence and have not seen any recent literature on the subject. Which is the single most appropriate response to give in this situation? ★

A Advise her that there is a financial penalty for practices if patients do not attend screening appointments, so she should make every effort to keep her appointment

B Agree with her that there are reasonable concerns about the benefits of mammography, and advise her not to take any further part in the screening programme

C Explain that you are not aware of the evidence that she has raised with you, so you are going to refer her to a specialist breast surgeon for up-to-date advice

D Explain that you are not aware of the evidence that she has raised with you, but that you could help her to interpret it once you have looked at it yourself

E Explain that you are not aware of the evidence that she has raised with you, so it is unlikely to be true and she should attend for screening

9. A 48-year-old woman has recently moved into the practice area. At her induction health check, the practice nurse notes that her weight is 85 kg and her height is 160 cm. Which single health factor would you consider in advising her about her weight? ★

A She is at increased risk of stomach cancer and needs to lose weight to a body mass index (BMI) of 25 kg/m² to bring her risk down to acceptable levels

B She is at increased risk of stomach cancer and needs to lose 20 kg to bring her risk down to acceptable levels

C She is at increased risk of hypertension and should lose 5 kg to bring her risk down to acceptable levels

D She is at increased risk of kidney stones and needs to lose 10 kg to bring her risk down to acceptable levels

E She is at increased risk of type 2 diabetes and should lose 20 kg to bring her risk down to acceptable levels

10. A 22-year-old student has muscle aches, malaise, headache, and anorexia that started 2 days ago. Today he has a temperature of 39.4°C. Which is the single most important direct question to ask him as part of history taking in order to confirm the likely diagnosis? ★

A Has he been bitten by an animal recently?

B Has he had close contact with anyone else with similar symptoms?

C Has he recently eaten any food that he thinks might have 'gone off'?

D Has he travelled overseas recently?

E Is he taking any medication at present?

11. A 55-year-old diabetic man asks for the vaccines he had last year against flu and pneumonia. His records show that he had the influenza and pneumococcal vaccines last year. Which is the single most appropriate piece of advice to give him? ★

A The influenza vaccine that he had last year will protect him against influenza for another 5 years

B He does not need another influenza vaccine this year but should have it next year

C He does not need another pneumococcal vaccine this year but should have it next year

D He is in a high-risk category for influenza and should have this vaccine every year

E He is in a high-risk category for pneumonia and influenza and should have both vaccines every year

12. A 50-year-old man with convictions for violence comes to the surgery reception, smelling of alcohol and demanding dihydrocodeine. Which is the single best way of managing this situation? ★

A Ask him to take a seat in the waiting room to be seen in order with the other patients

B Immediately show him to the next available doctor

C Phone the police and ask them to remove him

D Physically eject him from the premises and lock the surgery door

E Place him in a vacant room and ask a doctor to see him when they are available

13. An 84-year-old woman is in hospital recovering from a total hip replacement, following a fall in her flat. She was previously independent, despite living on the first floor, and drove her own car to the nearby shops. Who is the single best professional to ensure that she is safe to return to her flat? ★

A Age Concern worker

B General practitioner (GP)

C Health visitor

D Occupational therapist

E Physiotherapist

14. An 18-year-old man has a sore throat, fever, and malaise. A monospot test is sent and comes back positive. Which is the single most important element to avoid at this stage? ★

A Alcohol

B Contact sports

C Fatty foods

D Kissing

E Paracetamol

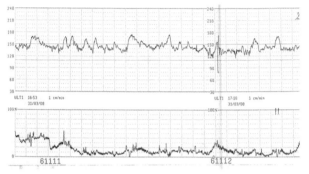

Figure 1.1

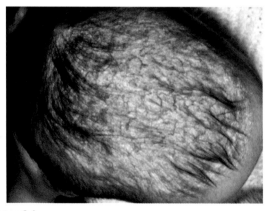

Figure 2.1
Courtesy of Barts and the London NHS Trust

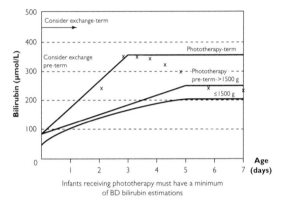

Figure 2.2

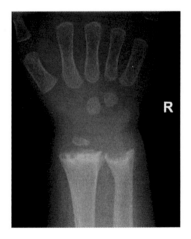

Figure 2.3

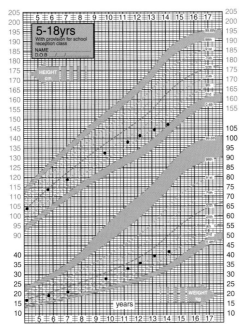

Figure 2.4

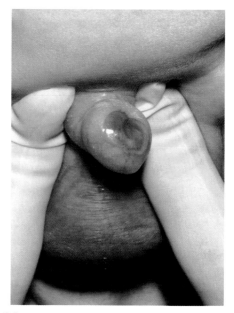

Figure 2.5

Reproduced with permission from Baldwin A, Hjelde N, Goumalatsou C, and Myers G, *Oxford Handbook of Clinical Specialties*, Tenth edition, figure 2.6, p. 132. Copyright (2017) with permission from Oxford University Press

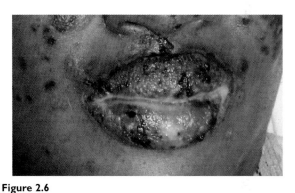

Figure 2.6
Courtesy of Barts and the London NHS Trust

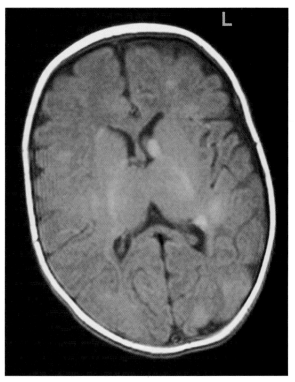

Figure 2.7

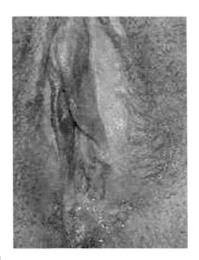

Figure 3.1

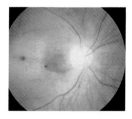

Figure 5.1

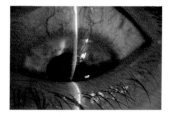

Figure 5.2

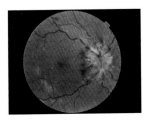

Figure 5.3

Courtesy of Masoud Teimory

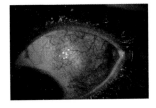

Figure 5.4

Reproduced with permission from Sundaram V, Barsam A, Barker L, Khaw PT, *Training in Ophthalmology*, Second edition, figure 7.36, p.271. Copyright (2016) with permission from Oxford University Press

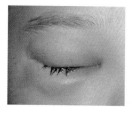

Figure 5.5

Reproduced with permission from Sundaram V, Barsam A, Alwitry A, Khaw PT, *Training in Ophthalmology*, First edition, Figure 10.8. Copyright (2009) with permission from Oxford University Press

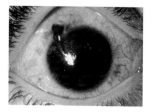

Figure 5.6

Reproduced with permission from Sundaram V, Barsam A, Barker L, Khaw PT, *Training in Ophthalmology*, Second edition, figure 2.82, p. 103. Copyright (2016) with permission from Oxford University Press

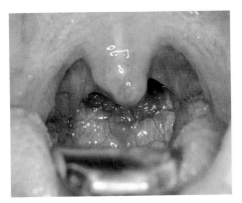

Figure 7.1

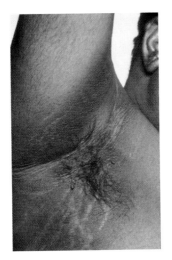

Figure 8.1
Courtesy of Barts and the London NHS Trust

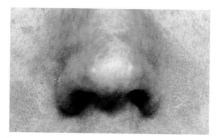

Figure 8.2
Courtesy of Barts and the London NHS Trust

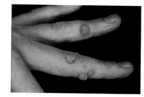

Figure 8.3
Courtesy of Barts and the London NHS Trust

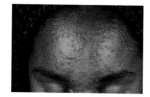

Figure 8.4
Courtesy of Barts and the London NHS Trust

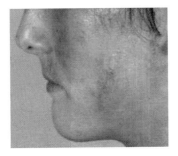

Figure 8.5
Courtesy of Barts and the London NHS Trust

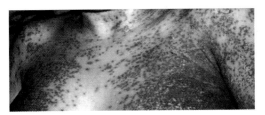

Figure 8.6
Courtesy of Barts and the London NHS Trust

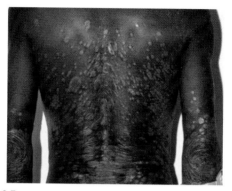

Figure 8.7
Courtesy of Barts and the London NHS Trust

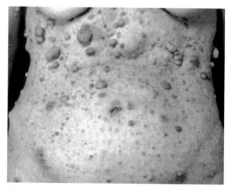

Figure 8.8
Courtesy of Barts and the London NHS Trust

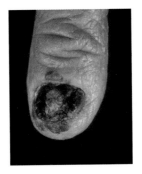

Figure 8.9
Courtesy of Barts and the London NHS Trust

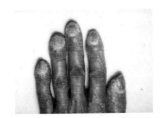

Figure 8.10
Courtesy of Barts and the London NHS Trust

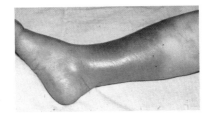

Figure 8.11
Courtesy of Barts and the London NHS Trust

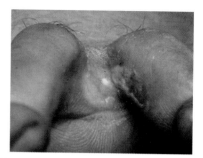

Figure 8.12
Courtesy of Barts and the London NHS Trust

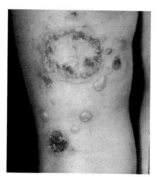

Figure 8.13
Courtesy of Barts and the London NHS Trust

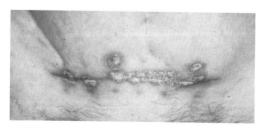

Figure 8.14
Courtesy of Barts and the London NHS Trust

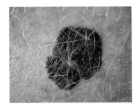

Figure 8.15
Courtesy of Barts and the London NHS Trust

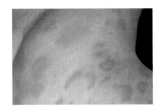

Figure 8.16
Courtesy of Barts and the London NHS Trust

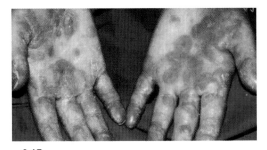

Figure 8.17
Courtesy of Barts and the London NHS Trust

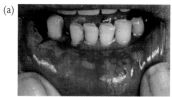

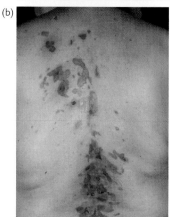

Figure 8.18
Courtesy of Barts and the London NHS Trust

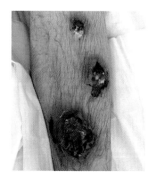

Figure 8.19
Courtesy of Barts and the London NHS Trust

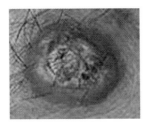

Figure 8.20
Courtesy of Barts and the London NHS Trust

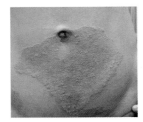

Figure 8.21
Courtesy of Barts and the London NHS Trust

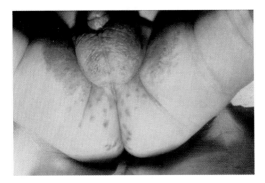

Figure 8.22
Courtesy of Barts and the London NHS Trust

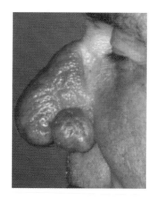

Figure 8.23
Courtesy of Barts and the London NHS Trust

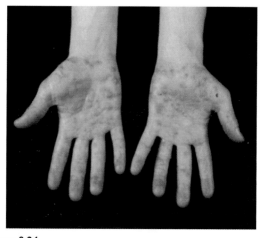

Figure 8.24
Courtesy of Barts and the London NHS Trust

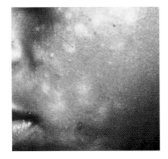

Figure 8.25
Courtesy of Barts and the London NHS Trust

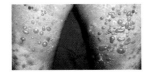

Figure 8.26
Courtesy of Barts and the London NHS Trust

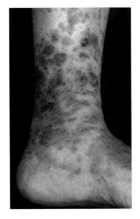

Figure 8.27
Courtesy of Barts and the London NHS Trust

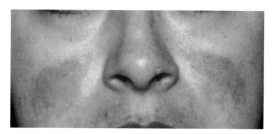

Figure 8.28
Courtesy of Barts and the London NHS Trust

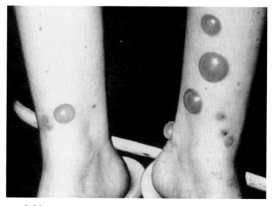

Figure 8.29
Courtesy of Barts and the London NHS Trust

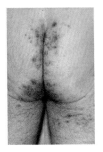

Figure 8.30
Courtesy of Barts and the London NHS Trust

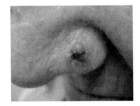

Figure 8.31
Courtesy of Barts and the London NHS Trust

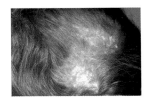

Figure 8.32
Courtesy of Barts and the London NHS Trust

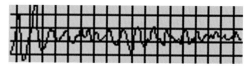

Figure 9.1

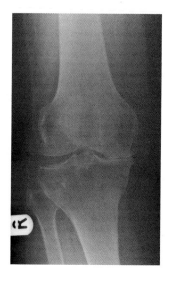

Figure 11.1

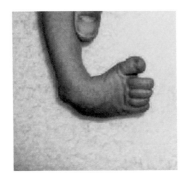

Figure 11.2

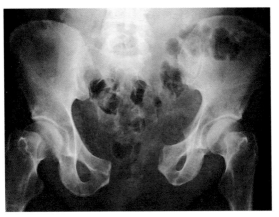

Figure 12.1

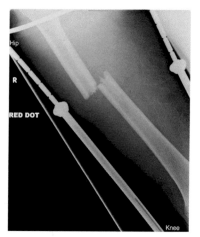

Figure 12.2

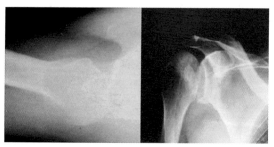

Figure 12.3

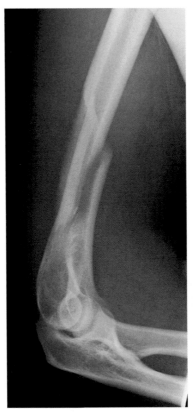

Figure 12.4

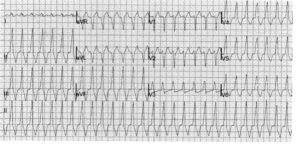

Figure 13.1

15. A 21-year-old student comes for a repeat prescription of her combined oral contraceptive pill (the Pill). She has been having bad one-sided headaches, with flashing lights lasting a few minutes prior to the headache since starting the Pill. She has a past history of migraine when stressed and has some exams coming up. Her blood pressure is 100/70 mmHg, and her clinical examination is normal. Which is the single most appropriate management? ★

A Advise her that the headaches are most probably caused by exam stress

B Advise her to stop taking the Pill if the flashing lights last longer than 60 minutes

C Stop the Pill she is taking, and try a different combined oral contraceptive pill

D Stop the Pill she is taking, and consider a progestogen-only pill instead

E Stop the Pill she is taking, and refer her urgently to a neurologist

16. A 65-year-old woman, who lives alone, has chronic knee pain and is prescribed a course of non-steroidal anti-inflammatory drugs (NSAIDs) for the first time. After she has left the surgery, you notice from her record that she is asthmatic. Which is the single most appropriate way to communicate to the patient not to take the medication? ★

A Ask the receptionist to make her a routine appointment for the next day

B Phone her and give her the appropriate advice

C Phone the local chemist and instruct them not to issue the prescription

D Phone the police and ask them to go to her house

E Write to her, requesting her to make an urgent appointment

17. A 21-year-old single mother has a 2-month-old baby who is not sleeping and seems perpetually hungry. She is still breastfeeding but thinks that she will have to change her baby to bottle-feeding. She wants some advice about this. Who is the single best person from the health-care team to advise her? ★

A District nurse

B General practitioner (GP)

C Health visitor

D Midwife

E Social worker

18. A 22-year-old woman has persistent headaches, nausea, and disturbed sleep and feels tired and cold all the time. She appears very thin, and her body mass index (BMI) is 16 kg/m². She tells you that this is the right weight for her. Which single health-care professional would it be most appropriate to refer her to? ★

A Continue to see her yourself as a general practitioner (GP)

B Dietitian

C Endocrinologist

D Neurologist

E Psychiatrist

19. A 32-year-old woman is 33 weeks pregnant with her second child. She has come for a routine antenatal appointment. During her first pregnancy, she had pre-eclampsia and required a hospital admission and early delivery. Today she is feeling tired and 'off colour'. Which single combination of clinical features would suggest that she could be suffering from pre-eclampsia requiring immediate hospital referral? ★

A Raised blood pressure alone

B Raised blood pressure and proteinuria

C Raised blood pressure, proteinuria, and headache

D Raised blood pressure, proteinuria, and peripheral oedema

E Raised blood pressure, proteinuria, and seizures

20. A 17-year-old man has had a sore throat, fever, malaise, and headache for 4 days. He has bilaterally enlarged tonsils with exudate, and cervical lymphadenopathy. Which single complication of his illness may be prevented by treatment with oral penicillin? ★

A Drug eruption

B Glomerulonephritis

C Mesenteric adenitis

D Otitis media

E Sinusitis

21. A 65-year-old woman with osteoarthritis affecting both knees is in need of some pain relief. However, she is unwilling to take anti-inflammatory drugs, as she says that they make her feel ill and other painkillers make her constipated. She asks whether there is anything other than standard painkillers that could help her pain. Which is the single most appropriate therapy to recommend? ★ ★

A Glucosamine and chondroitin

B Homeopathy

C Modern acupuncture using trigger points

D Reflexology

E Transcutaneous electrical nerve stimulation (TENS) machine

22. A man has a chest infection. He is prescribed a course of amoxicillin for 1 week. He also wants a repeat prescription of his blood pressure medication. Under which single circumstance is he eligible to obtain the medications without paying prescription charges for them? ★

A He earns less than £25 000 per annum

B He has a partner and more than three children at home

C He has been unwell for more than 4 weeks

D He has diabetes

E He is aged over 50 years

23. A 35-year-old woman is 12 weeks pregnant. She has significant dysuria, urinary frequency, and offensive-smelling urine. A dipstick test shows 3+ blood, 3+ leucocytes, and 2+ nitrites. Which single treatment regime is most appropriate? ★ ★

A Amoxicillin for 7 days

B Encourage oral fluids and simple analgesia

C Nalidixic acid for 7 days

D Nitrofurantoin for 7 days

E Trimethoprim for 3 days

24. A 36-year-old woman attends the surgery for her 'pill check'. She has been on the combined hormonal contraceptive (CHC) Microgynon® for 18 years and wants to continue it as she has had no problems with it. She smokes ten cigarettes a day. Her blood pressure is 140/88 mmHg, and her body mass index (BMI) is 30 kg/m². Which is the single most appropriate management? ★ ★

A Explain that her blood pressure is too high for the CHC and she needs to consider changing to an alternative method of contraception

B Explain that her BMI is too high for the CHC and she needs to consider changing to an alternative method of contraception

C Explain that she has an increased risk of ovarian cancer on the CHC and she needs to consider changing to an alternative method of contraception

D Explain that smoking increases the risks associated with the CHC and she needs to consider changing to an alternative method of contraception

E Give her a further prescription for Microgynon®, and arrange a review in 6 months

25. A 50-year-old man seeks advice about his father, who has mild dementia and is living in a nursing home. The father is becoming increasingly unwell with a chest infection, and the son wants him to be admitted to hospital, but the father wishes to stay where he is. Which is the single best summary of the legal situation? ★ ★

A As the father has dementia, he is not competent and therefore the son can and should decide on his treatment

B The father is competent and can therefore decide on his own treatment, regardless of the son's opinion

C The father is not competent and therefore decisions about his care must be made by his doctor, based on the patient's best interests

D The father's competence should be assessed and, if he has capacity, he can accept or decline treatment himself, regardless of the consequences

E The father's competence should be assessed, but his doctor may insist on admission, should his condition deteriorate, on the grounds of necessity

26. A 35-year-old woman with persistent irritable bowel syndrome asks to see a complementary therapist to help her with her symptoms. She understands that she may need to pay for this privately and that there may not be good evidence for the effectiveness of some complementary treatments, but she says that she is convinced that this is what she would like to do. Which is the single most appropriate action to take in response to her request? ★ ★

A Ask her to identify a practitioner whom she would like to see, and then provide a written referral if this is requested

B Decline to refer her on the grounds that this will avoid the need to pay private care fees

C Refer her directly to a colleague who runs a private complementary clinic

D Refer her to a gastroenterologist because she is more likely to achieve better symptom control with the help of a conventional specialist

E Refer her to a therapist selected from the Yellow Pages on the basis of geographical proximity to her home

27. A 65-year-old woman, who regularly attends with symptoms related to chronic depression, has some vague muscle ache and headache. She has been told before that her symptoms may well be related to her depression, but she requests further assessment. Which single aspect of her history is the most likely to point to a significant alternative diagnosis? ★ ★

A She has been experiencing pain in her hip when walking

B She has been experiencing some stinging pain on passing urine

C She has noticed a deterioration of her vision

D She has noticed some hearing loss in her left ear

E She has recently started taking herbal remedies for her depression

28. The local pharmacist has sent back a prescription written this morning. He says a controlled drug has been prescribed wrongly—a patient with intractable chronic back pain has been given a prescription for morphine modified release (MST Continus®). Which single element must be on a prescription for a controlled drug? ★ ★

A The date must be written in words and figures

B The diagnosis must be specified

C The full name and address of the patient must be handwritten, not typed

D The prescriber's General Medical Council registration number must be given

E The total quantity to dispense must be expressed in words and figures

29. A medical student is sitting in on a general practitioner (GP) surgery. One of the patients says that he would rather not have a student present. Which is the single most appropriate way of handling this? ★ ★ ★

A Before calling the patient in, ask the student to wait in another room

B Emphasize the importance of student teaching, hoping that the patient will reconsider

C Introduce the student and confirm that the patient would prefer the student to leave

D Rebook the patient for another surgery when you do not have students present

E Reschedule the patient to the end of surgery

30. A 62-year-old woman has had a unilateral painful rash, highly suggestive of shingles, for 36 hours. She asks if she could pass it on to her grandson, who is 7 days old. He lives in the same town and she last saw him yesterday. The baby's mother does not think she has ever had chickenpox. Which is the single most appropriate piece of advice to give to the grandmother? ★ ★ ★

A As the baby has been in contact with her, he should receive zoster immunoglobulin (ZIG) as soon as possible

B It is better to get chickenpox during childhood than later in life, and she need not worry about contact

C It is better to get shingles during childhood than later in life, and she need not worry about contact

D The baby could get chickenpox, and she should avoid seeing him until the blisters have crusted over

E The baby will be protected by maternal antibodies and will not be affected

31. A 50-year-old woman has hypertension and is on ramipril. She has dizziness, imbalance, and nausea. It can occur during the day or night, but she has noticed that it often happens when she looks up and she has had difficulty getting out of bed in the mornings. There are no headaches, visual symptoms, or any problems with her hearing. In surgery, she is not feeling dizzy. Her blood pressure (BP) is 116/70 mmHg, with no postural drop. Cranial nerve examination is normal, with normal speech and gait. There is no tremor, past pointing, or dysdiadochokinesia. Which is the single best course of action for this lady? ★ ★ ★

A Admit her to hospital for a head computed tomography (CT) scan

B Perform the Epley maneuvre

C Prescribe prochlorperazine 5 mg three times daily (TDS)

D Refer for vestibular rehabilitation exercises

E Stop her antihypertensive

32. A 40-year-old woman has heavy periods. Her periods have always been heavy, but now they are getting worse and she wants to discuss possible treatments. She has no inter-menstrual or post-coital bleeding, and she is up-to-date with her cervical smears. She is otherwise well, with no significant past medical history. She has two children and does not want any more. Her husband has had a vasectomy. Which is the single most appropriate management? ★ ★ ★ ★

A Arrange blood tests, including a full blood count, a thyroid and hormone profile, and a pelvic ultrasound scan

B Conduct a pelvic examination and offer insertion of the Mirena® coil

C Conduct a pelvic examination and offer the combined hormone contraceptive pill

D Refer her to gynaecology for consideration of endometrial ablation

E Refer her to gynaecology for consideration of hysterectomy

33. A 68-year-old man was watching television 10 days ago when his wife noticed that the right side of his face was drooping, his speech was slurred, and he could not move his right hand. This only lasted for 10 minutes, so he did not seek any medical help at the time. He has no other medical problems and is not on any medication. His blood pressure is 130/70 mmHg and examination is unremarkable. Which is the single most appropriate management? ★ ★ ★ ★

A Admit him to hospital, as he has had a transient ischaemic attack (TIA) and is at high risk of progression to having a stroke

B Commence 75 mg aspirin and arrange blood tests, including cholesterol and glucose

C Commence 75 mg aspirin and refer him routinely to a medical clinic for further investigations

D Commence 300 mg aspirin and refer him to a TIA clinic to be seen within 24 hours

E Commence 300 mg aspirin and refer him to a TIA clinic to be seen within 1 week

34. A 58-year-old man attends for his annual diabetic review. As well as diabetes, he has a history of a myocardial infarction (MI) 5 years ago, from which he recovered well. He now works as a delivery driver. In clinic, his body mass index (BMI) is 32 kg/m², blood pressure (BP) 126/70 mmHg, and a urine dipstick shows protein 1+ and blood 2+. His recent blood results show:

- HbA1c 68 mmol/mol
- glomerular filtration rate (GFR) 54 mL/min/1.73 m² (stable)
- liver function tests (LFTs) normal
- full blood count (FBC) normal

His current medications are ramipril 10 mg once daily (OD), metformin 1 g twice daily (BD), aspirin 75 mg OD, and atorvastatin 80 mg OD. He has been advised on optimizing his lifestyle. Which is the single most appropriate step in improving his diabetic control?

A Refer to the local diabetic clinic for consideration of insulin therapy

B Start a dipeptidylpeptidase-4 inhibitor such as sitagliptin

C Start a sodium–glucose co-transporter-2 (SGLT2) inhibitor such as canagliflozin

D Start a sulfonylurea such as gliclazide

E Start a thiazolidinedione such as pioglitazone

ANSWERS

1. C ★

The BMI is calculated as weight in kilograms divided by height in metres squared (kg/m^2). It is a measure of weight for height and does not represent body fat or other ratios.

2. A ★   OHCS 10th edn → p. 672

Retention of urine and faeces should raise suspicions of cauda equina syndrome (compression of the cauda equina in the spinal canal). Pain and inability to perform a straight leg raise can be caused by muscular back injury or sciatica, and ankle jerks are usually brisk in cord compression.

→ http://patient.info/doctor/low-back-pain-and-sciatica

→ http://cks.nice.org.uk/sciatica-lumbar-radiculopathy

3. C ★

All competent patients have a right to confidentiality, and you should not break this unless the patient specifically gives consent for you to share the information. However, if the mother wants to express her concerns about her daughter, it is acceptable to listen to these without revealing any information.

→ http://www.gmc-uk.org/guidance/ethical_guidance/confidentiality.asp

4. E ★

There are several risk factors for stroke, some of which can be modified and some of which cannot. Hypertension is considered to be an important risk factor for stroke, with well-documented relationships between blood pressure and the occurrence of stroke. There is also good evidence that treating hypertension reduces the risk of stroke. Atrial fibrillation is the most important risk factor for stroke, being that atrial fibrillation increases the risk of stroke by 480% (hypertension by 140%). However, there is no mention that this man is in atrial fibrillation.

5. C ★   OHCS 10th edn → p. 480

An approach that is patient-centred and which identifies, acknowledges, and respects the patient's decisions and feelings ensures a better long-term result. It is important to realize that all patients have different life factors that may influence their decision-making. Respecting these is vital for building a lasting relationship.

6. D ★   OHCS 10th edn → p. 515

All of these are possible risk factors for poor sleep, apart from moderate cigarette smoking. However, the suggestion of low mood and possible depression is an important presenting symptom that needs to be followed up.

7. E ★   OHCS 10th edn → p. 273

HPV can cause cervical abnormalities that may progress to become cancer. There are hundreds of HPVs, of which types 16 and 18 cause 70% of HPV-related cervical cancers. HPV types 6 and 11 are associated with genital warts. In the UK, two vaccines are currently used. Cervarix® immunizes against types 16 and 18, and Gardasil® immunizes against types 6, 11, 16, and 18. The current programme schedule involves three doses given at 0, 1–2, and 6 months. The Department of Health recommends that any women under the age of 18 years with unknown or incomplete immunization status should complete the course. Those from overseas who are not protected should be offered protection.

→ https://www.gov.uk/government/publications/human-papillomavirus-hpv-the-green-book-chapter-18a

8. D ★

A common-sense approach to difficult situations such as this that respects the main principles of patient autonomy, beneficence, and non-maleficence is needed here. General practitioners may have to help patients to interpret health information, especially now that they have access to so much more information via the Internet.

9. E ★   OHCS 10th edn → p. 514

Type 2 diabetes is greatly increased in overweight people and is a major cause of morbidity. A healthy BMI is in the range of 20–25 kg/m². If this woman lost 20 kg, her weight would be 65 kg. Her BMI would therefore be $65/1.6^2$, which is 25.4 kg/m². This is a much healthier BMI and an achievable range to aim for.

→ http://www.nice.org.uk/guidance/cg43

10. D ★

A possible diagnosis is malaria, which would be suspected if the patient had travelled to a region where malaria is prevalent.

11. D ★

The influenza vaccine is prepared each year from viruses of the three strains that are thought most likely to cause flu that winter. It is about 70% effective, and protection lasts for 1 year. Pneumococcal vaccine only needs to be given once. Both are recommended for high-risk groups of patients, including individuals with diabetes.

→ http://www.gov.uk/government/publications/influenza-the-green-book-chapter-19
→ http://www.gov.uk/government/publications/pneumococcal-the-green-book-chapter-25

12. **E** ★

Although all patients are entitled to appropriate treatment, you should not place other patients or practice staff at risk of harm. This patient has the same right to treatment as do others, but you should not disadvantage other patients by seeing him first simply because he is demanding. It may be necessary to call the police, but you may well be able to advise and treat him without difficulty, and you should endeavour to do this before taking more drastic action.

13. **D** ★

The occupational therapist's role is to assess patients with regard to their activities of daily living and to advise on how to make these activities achievable.

14. **B** ★

Glandular fever, or infectious mononucleosis, caused by Epstein–Barr virus, can cause splenomegaly. A rare, but serious, complication is splenic rupture, the risk of which is increased by contact sports and trauma to the area. The splenomegaly usually lasts for 6 to 8 weeks.

15. **D** ★   OHCS 10th edn → p. 300

The Pill can increase the risk of ischaemic stroke. Women who have a history of migraine should stop the Pill immediately if they develop aura and worsening headache, and they should have an ischaemic event excluded if these symptoms persist. The progestogen-only pill is a safe alternative, as it contains no oestrogen, which is the component that leads to the increased risk.

→ http://www.bnf.org/bnf (see Section 7.3.1; requires registration)

→ http://www.fsrh.org/standards-and-guidance/documents/combined-hormonal-contraception

16. **B** ★

NSAIDs may cause worsening of asthma, although this is not always the case. However, the patient should be warned about the risk and advised not to take the medication. The most effective way to ensure that this is done is to speak to her yourself. A further appointment can be offered to discuss alternative treatments later.

17. **C** ★   OHCS 10th edn → p. 472

The health visitor is a qualified nurse with a health visiting qualification (which includes public health nursing and health promotion). She takes over home visiting of new mothers from the midwife when the baby is 10 days old.

18. E ★   OHCS 10th edn → p. 382

There is a high probability that this woman has anorexia nervosa. She has symptoms of underweight and starvation, a persistently low BMI below 17 kg/m², and a belief that this is the right weight despite symptoms. She needs to be assessed and managed by an eating disorders specialist team, led by a psychiatrist, as part of mental health services. You may of course continue to see her as a GP, but she needs specialist help to direct her treatment.

19. C ★   OHCS 10th edn → p. 48

Pre-eclampsia is defined as hypertension plus proteinuria, with or without peripheral oedema. However, the presence of symptoms such as headache makes hospital referral important here. The presence of seizures would make the diagnosis eclampsia, rather than pre-eclampsia.

20. B ★

Although there is no clear evidence to support the use of antibiotics to reduce the incidence of post-streptococcal glomerulonephritis, antibiotics are often given in primary care for this reason.

21. E ★★

Many patients seek complementary therapies and alternative to prescribed medicines, so it is useful to have some idea of these. Initial trials for glucosamine showed some improvement in osteoarthritis; however, these were using different preparations which are not available to the public, and more recent trials have shown no benefits. The National Institute for Health and Care Excellence (NICE) does not recommend glucosamine for osteoarthritis. NICE does state that TENS machines should be offered as an adjunct in the treatment of osteoarthritis.

→ http://pathways.nice.org.uk/pathways/osteoarthritis

22. D ★

This patient would qualify for free prescriptions if he was aged over 60 years and if he had a low income and less than £16 000 in savings or investments, or if he had one of a number of chronic diseases. Help is based on a comparison between an individual's weekly income and assessed requirements at the time when the claim is made (or the date on which the charge was paid if a refund is claimed).

→ http://www.nhsbsa.nhs.uk/healthcosts

23. D ★★

This patient clearly has a significant urinary tract infection and needs antibiotic treatment. Trimethoprim and nalidixic acid are contraindicated in the first trimester of pregnancy, and amoxicillin, although safe, is likely to be ineffective due to widespread resistance. Nitrofurantoin is safe in early pregnancy but is best avoided near term, because of the possible risk of haemolytic anaemia in newborn babies.

24. D ★★   OHCS 10th edn → p. 300

When re-prescribing 'the Pill', the blood pressure and BMI should be re-corded, as well as the smoking history and whether the patient is having any problems. A smoking history is important because both smoking and the oral CHC can increase the risk of venous thromboembolism. The cut-off age for prescribing the Pill in a smoker is 35 years. There is no evidence that a lower-strength pill decreases this risk. Although this woman's BMI is raised and she is obese, the cut-off BMI for prescribing the Pill is 35 kg/m^2. CHC use may be associated with a small increase in the risk of cervical cancer, which is related to duration of use, and a small increased risk of breast cancer, which will reduce with time after stop-ping, but a reduced risk of ovarian and endometrial cancer that continues for several decades after stopping. A persistently raised blood pressure over 160/95 mmHg would mean that this patient should stop the Pill and consider an alternative, which could include a progesterone-only pill, depot, or implant, or an intrauterine device (IUD) or intrauterine system (IUS).

→ http://www.fsrh.org/standards-and-guidance/documents/combined-hormonal-contraception

25. D ★★   OHCS 10th edn → p. 409

The patient may have capacity, but it needs to be assessed. If he is com-petent, he can refuse or accept any treatment that is offered. However, he cannot insist on treatment that is not considered appropriate by his doctor. This legal situation is covered by different Acts in England and Wales, and in Scotland.

26. A ★★

Provided that you are happy that the patient is not at risk of harm, it is appropriate to facilitate a referral to a complementary therapist if they request it. However, because this is a private referral, you need to ensure that it is done professionally, that the patient has as much choice as possible, and that there is no suggestion that you have a personal interest in the referral.

27. C ★★

A wide variety of symptoms can occur in depression. However, it is important always to revisit the diagnosis and to assess every pres-entation fully. In an elderly woman with headaches and myalgia, loss of vision may occur in giant cell arteritis, and prompt treatment can save sight.

28. E ★★

Prescriptions for controlled drugs must be indelible and include:

- the name and address of the patient
- the form and strength of the preparation
- the total quantity in both words and figures of the preparation, or the number in both words and figures of dosage units, to be supplied
- the dose to be given
- the prescriber's name, signature, and address
- the date of the prescription.

Pharmacists cannot dispense, unless the prescription is filled in correctly.

→ http://www.bnf.org (requires registration)

29. A ★★★

When asking a patient whether they will allow a student to be present, you should have an appropriate mechanism to ensure that this does not pressurize the patient, embarrass either them or the student, or disadvantage the patient in any way.

30. A ★★★   OHCS 10th edn → p. 144

Neonates with significant exposure to chickenpox or shingles should receive ZIG as soon as possible. The fact that the mother has probably never had chickenpox means that she has no varicella antibodies to pass across the placenta, and the baby therefore has no protection.

31. B ★★★   OHCS 10th edn → pp. 554–5

This lady has benign paroxysmal positional vertigo (BPPV). This is the commonest vestibular disorder seen in primary care. It is provoked by certain movements of the head, such as looking up or rolling over and getting out of bed. It can be associated with nausea, but not usually vomiting, and patients are well in between episodes. BPPV can settle without treatment but may last a long time. Repositioning manoeuvres, such as the Epley manoeuvre, are more effective than vestibular suppressant medication, which should not be used long term. If this lady's symptoms persist and are debilitating, it may be appropriate to refer her to a specialist clinic, but trials of simple treatment should be done first.

→ https://cks.nice.org.uk/benign-paroxysmal-positional-vertigo
→ http://www.gpnotebook.co.uk/

32. B ★★★★   OHCS 10th edn → p. 250

The National Institute for Health and Care Excellence (NICE) has provided guidelines on the management of heavy periods. These suggest that in simple heavy menstrual bleeding, the only investigation required is a full blood count to rule out anaemia. A pelvic examination is only required if a structural or histological abnormality is suspected or an intrauterine device is being considered. The first-line recommended treatment is a Mirena® coil, with treatments such as non-steroidal anti-inflammatory drugs, tranexamic acid, and combined hormone contraceptives being second-line treatment. Surgical management is considered if pharmaceutical treatments have failed and/or there is a severe impact on the woman's quality of life, after full discussion of the risks.

→ https://pathways.nice.org.uk/pathways/heavy-menstrual-bleeding

33. E ★★★★

A TIA is defined as stroke symptoms and signs that resolve within 24 hours. Patients who present with a TIA need to be assessed to determine whether they are at high or low risk, using the validated ABCD^2 (Age, Blood pressure, Clinical features, Duration of symptoms, and Diabetes) tool. A patient with an ABCD^2 score higher than 4 is at high risk and should have specialist assessment and investigations, such as cholesterol and carotid Dopplers, within 24 hours. Patients with a score of 3 or less or who present more than 1 week after the event should have specialist assessment and investigation within 1 week. This man has a score of 3 and is therefore at lower risk. All patients should be started on 300 mg aspirin, unless this is contraindicated.

34. B ★★★★

This gentleman is obese, has chronic kidney disease stage 3 (CKD3) and established cardiovascular disease (CVD). His occupation is driving, so he needs to avoid hypoglycaemic attacks. A dipeptidylpeptidase-4 inhibitor, such as sitagliptin, would be the most appropriate option here, as it is weight-neutral and safe to be used in all stages of CKD and with established CVD. It also carries a low risk of hypoglycaemia. SGLT2 inhibitors are not licensed for initiation with a GFR less than 60. Sulfonylureas cause weight gain, carry a risk of hypoglycaemia, and can increase the risk of cardiovascular death. Pioglitazone can also cause significant weight gain and has been associated with bladder cancer, so this man's haematuria would need to be fully investigated before commencing pioglitazone.

→ http://pathways.nice.org.uk/pathways/type-2-diabetes-in-adults

Chapter 7

ENT

Philippa Tostevin

Ear, nose, and throat (ENT) surgery is a fascinating specialty. It is involved in the diagnosis and management of a vast range of diseases presenting from birth through all ages. The pathologies covered range from congenital airway obstruction in the neonate to head and neck malignancies in the elderly. Systemic diseases can also manifest for the first time in the ENT area. The creation of a surgical airway in the form of a tracheostomy can be lifesaving, but some ENT surgery is performed to improve quality of life, so it is particularly important to understand the indications for surgical interventions. In contrast to other surgical specialties, many of the patients who are seen in the outpatient setting do not need surgery and medical management is required.

For those interested in ENT surgery as a career, there are different areas within this diverse field that can be followed to a specialist level. These include rhinology, otology, and neuro-otology, in addition to the specialist areas of paediatric ENT, head and neck cancer surgery, voice, and facial plastic surgery.

A thorough knowledge and understanding of the diagnosis and management of common ENT conditions is vital for those who wish to work in general practice, paediatrics, or emergency medicine. ENT conditions in children represent a very large proportion of the workload in any general practice setting. Various foreign bodies can be swallowed, inhaled, or inserted into the nose or ear, so an understanding of how and when these need to be removed is essential for any junior doctor working in the Emergency Department.

In this chapter, the questions are based on the important knowledge that needs to be accrued as an undergraduate or a recently qualified doctor, as many readers may not have the opportunity to work as a junior doctor in an ENT team before treating ENT patients in the Emergency Department or in a general practice setting.

QUESTIONS

1. A 78-year-old man has sudden onset of hoarse voice. He has a weak cough and he coughs when eating. He has been a smoker since the age of 18 years. He has a right-sided vocal cord palsy. Which is the single most likely anatomical site for his primary malignancy? ★

A Bronchus

B Larynx

C Oesophagus

D Oral cavity

E Parotid

2. A 32-year-old lorry driver has had a painless, discharging left ear for 10 years. His Weber's test lateralizes to the left. His Rinne's test is negative on the left and positive on the right. The external auditory meatus is filled with mucopurulent debris. Which is the single most likely diagnosis? ★

A Chronic otitis externa

B Chronic secretory otitis media

C Chronic suppurative otitis media

D Malignant otitis externa

E Middle ear effusion

3. A 66-year-old man has unilateral, non-pulsatile tinnitus that is keeping him awake at night. His pure-tone audiogram shows asymmetrical sensorineural hearing loss. Which single benign tumour may be responsible for these findings? ★

A Astrocytoma

B Glioma

C Meningioma

D Pleomorphic adenoma

E Vestibular schwannoma

4. A 76-year-old woman has right-sided otalgia and vertigo. Her Rinne's test is positive in both ears, and her Weber's test lateralizes to the left ear. There are vesicles present on the superior aspect of her right pinna and drooping of her face on the right side. Which single virus is most likely to have caused this clinical presentation? ★

A Adenovirus

B Cytomegalovirus

C Epstein–Barr virus

D Herpes simplex virus

E Varicella-zoster virus

5. A 23-year-old man has a 2-cm ulcer in his oral cavity. He has lost 3 kg in weight over the last 3 months. The edge of the ulcer is biopsied, and the histopathology result shows non-caseating granulomata. Which is the single most likely diagnosis? ★

A Actinomycosis

B Crohn's disease

C Tuberculosis

D Ulcerative colitis

E Vitamin B_{12} deficiency

6. A 23-year-old woman has had a fall at the gym. She now has a transient sensation of movement when she turns her head to the right. There is no hearing loss or tinnitus. Which is the single most likely diagnosis? ★

A Benign paroxysmal positional vertigo

B Labyrinthitis

C Ménière's disease

D Temporal bone fracture

E Vestibular neuronitis

7. A 17-year-old boy has sudden-onset hearing loss after standing near an exploding firework. He has a central perforation of the tympanic membrane and a conductive hearing loss. Which is the single most appropriate acute management? ★

A Emergency myringoplasty

B Grommet insertion

C Intravenous antibiotics

D Keep the ear dry and review

E Topical antibiotic and steroid drops

8. A 26-year-old man has had a foul-smelling, painless otorrhoea and a conductive hearing loss for 3 years. There is moist white debris in the attic of the right tympanic membrane. Which is the single most appropriate next intervention? ★

A Daily suction toilet

B Intravenous antibiotics

C Mastoid exploration

D Myringoplasty

E Ventilation tube insertion

9. A 63-year-old man has otalgia and a hard, craggy mass on the right tonsil. He has been a smoker for the last 40 years. Which is the single most likely histological type of tumour? ★

A Adenocarcinoma

B Lymphoma

C Rhabdomyosarcoma

D Small-cell carcinoma

E Squamous cell carcinoma

10. A 75-year-old woman has had a hoarse voice, lethargy, and weight gain for 8 weeks. On examination, her vocal cords appear thickened. Which single blood test is most likely to be helpful in making a diagnosis? ★

A Full blood count

B Liver function test

C Serum calcium level

D Thyroid function test

E Urea and electrolytes

11. A 3-year-old girl is snoring so loudly that she is keeping the family awake. She has never had tonsillitis, but an overnight sleep study has shown desaturations to 80% in room air when she is asleep. The oropharyngeal examination is shown in Figure 7.1 (see Colour Plate section). Which is the single most appropriate management strategy? ★

A Adenotonsillectomy

B Continuous home oxygen at night

C Continuous positive airway pressure (CPAP) via a face mask at night

D Palatal stiffening procedure

E Tonsillectomy

12. A 63-year-old diabetic man has an intensely itchy and painful right ear. Spores are seen in the external auditory meatus, which are cleared with microsuction. Which is the single most appropriate management? ★

A Aluminium acetate ear drops

B Glycerine and ichthammol

C Intravenous voriconazole

D Oral ketoconazole

E Topical clotrimazole

13. A 2-year-old boy has a temperature of 39°C and purulent otorrhoea. His pinna is laterally and inferiorly displaced, but the post-auricular sulcus is maintained. Which is the single most appropriate first-line emergency management strategy? ★

A Admit the patient for analgesia and observation

B Admit the patient for intravenous antibiotics

C Emergency grommet insertion

D Give antibiotic ear drops

E Give oral antibiotics

14. A 70-year-old man has had an intermittently discharging ear for 5 years. He has come for review. Which single new clinical finding would indicate that he may have developed a malignancy? ★

A Black spores in the external auditory meatus

B Circumferential oedema of the external auditory meatus

C Offensive-smelling discharge

D Purulent discharge

E Sanguineous discharge

15. A 20-year-old man has chronic facial pain and rhinorrhoea. He has had multiple courses of antibiotics, with little improvement in his symptoms. A coronal computed tomography (CT) scan of his paranasal sinuses shows a round opacity with mixed density within the right maxillary sinus. Which is the single most likely explanation for these findings? ★ ★

A Allergic polyp

B Angiofibroma

C Antrochoanal polyp

D Fungal ball

E Foreign body within the sinus

16. A 4-year-old boy with Down's syndrome has a proven middle ear effusion bilaterally that has been present for 6 months. His pure-tone hearing thresholds are 40 dB bilaterally. Which is the single most appropriate management? ★ ★

A Adenoidectomy

B Bilateral mastoidectomy

C Bilateral ventilation tube insertion

D Cochlea implantation

E Watch and wait for 3 months

17. A 68-year-old woman has otalgia and dysphagia. She has angular cheilitis and pale conjunctivae. Her oropharyngeal examination is normal. In which single anatomical site is this patient likely to have a tumour? ★ ★

A Lower oesophagus

B Nasopharynx

C Post-cricoid

D Thyroid

E Tonsil

18. A 47-year-old woman has pulsatile tinnitus in her right ear. Her hearing is normal. There is a red lesion visible on the promontory in the middle ear behind the tympanic membrane. Which is the single most likely diagnosis? ★ ★

A Arteriovenous malformation

B Carotid body tumour

C Glomus tumour

D Middle ear polyp

E Otosclerosis

19. A 72-year-old woman with rheumatoid arthritis has hoarseness of her voice. There is a left vocal cord palsy. Which single joint is likely to be involved? ★ ★

A Atlanto-occipital

B Cricoarytenoid

C Cricothyroid

D Costochondral

E Sternoclavicular

20. A 32-year-old woman is having intermittent episodes of vertigo. Each episode lasts for up to 12 hours, with associated tinnitus and hearing loss. Which single medication may be of help in reducing the frequency of her vertiginous episodes? ★★

A Amitriptyline

B Betahistine

C Cyclizine

D Paroxetine

E Prochlorperazine

21. A 2-year-old girl had an episode of acute otitis media 3 weeks ago. She now has no pain or temperature but has a residual hearing loss. A type B tympanometry trace is found, with a normal canal volume measurement. Which is the single most likely explanation for this result? ★★

A Cholesteatoma

B Chronic suppurative otitis media

C Perforation of the tympanic membrane

D Persistent acute otitis media

E Serous middle ear effusion

22. You are on a mountaineering expedition, far from medical help, and your colleague develops difficulty breathing, with cyanosis. You are unable to resuscitate him with rescue breaths and realize that a surgical airway is required to save his life. Which single anatomical structure would you locate and enter to access his airway in this situation?

A Cricoid ring

B Cricothyroid membrane

C Third tracheal ring

D Thyrohyoid membrane

E Thyroid cartilage

23. A 5-year-old boy has a submandibular lump. It is non-tender, with a light purplish discoloration of the overlying skin. He is apyrexial and otherwise well. His general practitioner (GP) has tried several courses of antibiotics, but the lump has continued to grow. Which is the single most likely diagnosis? ★★

A Atypical mycobacterial infection

B Brucellosis

C Infectious mononucleosis

D Lymphoma

E Toxoplasmosis

24. A 76-year-old man has acute disabling vertigo, with nausea and vomiting. He has no tinnitus and has normal hearing. He has an intention tremor. Which single test would be most helpful in establishing a diagnosis? ★★

A Audiogram

B Brainstem-evoked response testing

C Caloric testing

D Computed tomography (CT) scan of the brain

E Otoacoustic emissions

25. A 47-year-old opera singer presented to the ear, nose, and throat (ENT) clinic with loss of vocal range. Nasendoscopic examination revealed bilateral vocal cord nodules. Which single initial treatment option should be offered to this patient? ★★

A Laser ablation of the nodule

B Microdebridement of the nodule

C Propranolol

D Sharp dissection of the nodule

E Voice therapy

26. A 3-year-old child presents with periorbital oedema and chemosis. Her right eye is proptosed and the eye movement is restricted. Which is the single most appropriate imaging technique to reveal any subperiosteal abscess formation in the orbit? ★★★

A Computed tomography (CT) angiogram

B CT scan

C Magnetic resonance imaging (MRI) scan

D Ultrasound scan

E Sinus X-ray

27. A 2-year-old boy was playing with a small plastic toy and then began coughing for 2 minutes. His mother called 999. He is now completely well and eating and drinking normally, but the toy is nowhere to be found. Which is the single most appropriate initial management? ★★★

A Computed tomography (CT) scan of the chest

B Flexible oesophagogastroduodenoscopy

C Microlaryngoscopy and bronchoscopy

D Nasendoscopy in the Emergency Department

E Rigid oesophagoscopy

28. A 23-year-old woman has fallen from a tree onto her face. She has a nasal fracture and clear rhinorrhoea. The nasal discharge is positive for glucose. Which single test would you ask for to confirm the nature of the nasal fluid? ★ ★ ★

A Albumin

B β-galactosidase

C β-2 transferrin

D Ferritin

E Myoglobin

29. A 16-year-old boy sustains a nasal fracture during a game of football. He feels that his nose is obstructed. Both nasal bones are in the midline, and both nasal airways are obscured by red swollen mucosa, which is soft when palpated. Which is the single most appropriate initial management? ★ ★ ★

A Incision and drainage

B Manipulation of the nasal fracture

C Oral antibiotics and review

D Rhinoplasty

E Septoplasty

30. At 7 p.m., a 3-year-old girl is brought to the Emergency Department, having pushed a lithium battery up her nose earlier in the afternoon. It cannot be removed in the department. She last ate at 4 p.m. Which is the single most appropriate time to list her for removal of the battery under general anaesthetic? ★ ★ ★

A After a course of steroids to decrease the inflammation

B After waiting a few days for the inflammation to subside

C On the next available elective list

D This evening, as soon as possible

E Tomorrow morning once adequately fasted

31. A 47-year-old man presents to the general practitioner (GP) with a left-sided lower motor neurone facial palsy and an insidiously developing dysphagia. On oral examination, the doctor notices that the uvula is deviated to the right. The patient is apyrexial and otherwise appears well and is not in pain. What is the single most likely diagnosis?

A Deep lobe of a parotid tumour

B Glomus tumour

C Lymphoma of the tonsil

D Retropharyngeal abscess

E Quinsy

32. Following his laryngectomy operation, a 74-year-old man has his speech restored using a valve in a tracheo-oesophageal fistula. The speech therapist wishes to explain to him the mechanism whereby he is able to communicate again. Which is the single best description of the mechanism for his post-laryngectomy speech restoration? ★★★★

A A hand-held resonating device is used in conjunction with the valve to create speech

B A fenestrated tracheostomy tube is fitted to enable speech restoration

C Air from the lungs is diverted through the valve and up to the pharynx, which vibrates to create sound

D Air from the lungs is diverted through the valve, which vibrates to create sound

E Air is taken into the oesophagus, and this causes the valve to vibrate

33. A 37-year-old man has an epistaxis that has not been controlled with 24 hours of nasal packing and bed rest. His blood pressure is 120/72 mmHg. A decision to perform arterial ligation is made. Which single artery is most commonly ligated first in this situation? ★★★★

A External carotid

B Greater palatine

C Maxillary

D Posterior ethmoid

E Sphenopalatine

ANSWERS

1. B ★

About one-third of recurrent laryngeal nerve palsies are caused by cancers, and 40% of these are in the larynx. The risk is increased in smokers. The left recurrent laryngeal nerve has a long course and loops down under the arch of the aorta in the chest, so it may be affected in malignant tumours of the mediastinum. This is less common on the right side. Oesophageal cancers can have pressure effects, but dysphagia would be more prominent.

2. C ★   OHCS 10th edn → p. 544

There is a long history of suppuration here. Chronic suppurative otitis media causes a conductive hearing loss, demonstrated by the tuning fork tests. Otitis externa does not cause mucoid discharge, as the external ear canal does not produce mucus.

3. E ★   OHCS 10th edn → p. 553

A schwannoma, or acoustic neuroma, is a slow-growing benign tumour that causes problems by exerting local pressure on the eighth cranial nerve, which can result in tinnitus and hearing loss. The main differential diagnosis is a meningioma. However, in this location, vestibular schwannomas are commoner, although magnetic resonance imaging is needed to distinguish them.

4. E ★   OHCS 10th edn → p. 652

This is Ramsay Hunt syndrome, caused by reactivation of varicella-zoster virus in a patient who has had chickenpox in the past. The combination of otalgia, hearing impairment, vertigo, a lower motor neurone facial nerve palsy, and visible vesicles gives the diagnosis.

5. B ★

Crohn's disease causes non-caseating granulomata in the gastrointestinal (GI) tract anywhere from the mouth to the anus. It should always be a differential diagnosis in any patient with unusual or persistent mouth ulceration, especially when coupled with other GI signs or symptoms. Tuberculosis causes caseating granulomata. Ulcerative colitis affects only the colon, not the upper GI tract.

6. A ★   OHCS 10th edn → pp. 554–5

Benign positional vertigo is common after a head injury. Attacks are provoked by head movement. Labyrinthitis usually follows a viral illness. In Ménière's disease, there is associated tinnitus. Temporal bone fracture causes severe dizziness, often associated with facial nerve palsy and hearing loss.

7. D ★

Perforations may heal on their own, but while the drum is perforated, there is an increased risk of ear infection, so it is best to keep water out. Sudden loud noises may cause perforations, and surgical closure by means of a myringoplasty operation may be needed later.

8. C ★ OHCS 10th edn → p. 544

This man has a cholesteatoma—an area of skin in the middle ear that is locally destructive. It can be secondary to a tear in the tympanic membrane, followed by skin growing through. It should be considered if a patient has chronic discharge. On examination, a cottage cheese-like discharge is seen. If left untreated, it can invade intracranially, so surgical treatment is needed to remove the sac. A mastoidectomy may be required.

9. E ★ OHCS 10th edn → p. 572

Around 85% of pharyngeal cancers are squamous. Risk factors are smoking or chewing tobacco and older age. Human papillomavirus infection is an increasingly common cause.

10. D ★ OHCS 10th edn → p. 568

Hypothyroidism can cause oedema of the vocal cords, and therefore hoarseness. The history of lethargy and weight gain adds further clues. Thyroid dysfunction can also cause hoarseness due to pressure from a goitre. The list of causes of hoarseness is long, and therefore you need to look for other clues in the history and examination.

11. A ★

Airway obstruction due to tonsillar hypertrophy is an indication for tonsillectomy. This child's saturations are dipping to 80% during sleep, which indicates significant obstruction. Adenoid and tonsil tissue can be large in young children, and in this situation, both need to be removed. Although a Cochrane review has highlighted the fact that there are no good-quality trial data on efficacy, this is still the gold standard treatment when obstruction is demonstrated. If this fails and there are other problems such as significant obesity or neuromuscular disease, oxygen and CPAP may become necessary, but they are not first-line approaches to management. Similarly, palatal stiffening procedures, such as the insertion of implants, may be used in adults but are not appropriate in growing children.

→ http://www.cochrane.org/CD011165/ENT_tonsillectomy-or-without-adenoidectomy-versus-no-surgery-obstructive-sleep-disordered-breathing

12. E ★

Spores indicate a fungal infection, so an antifungal medication is needed. People who are immunocompromised are at increased risk of such infections. However, oral and intravenous treatments are not usually necessary as a first-line treatment, and topical treatment should be given in healthy patients. Aluminium acetate can be used as an astringent for otitis externa, but antifungal agents would be better in this proven fungal case.

13. B ★   OHCS 10th edn → p. 545

The high fever, thick purulent discharge, and distorted ear suggest mastoiditis. The ear is typically displaced laterally and inferiorly, and there may be swelling seen over the mastoid process behind the ear. This is a serious infection, and the child should be admitted and given intravenous antibiotics while surgical treatment is considered. Depending on the degree of damage, different surgical procedures are used to drain the pus.

14. E ★

Bloody discharge indicates a squamous cell carcinoma. The tumour tissue is friable and can bleed easily on contact.

15. D ★★   OHCS 10th edn → p. 558

In any patient with chronic recurrent sinus problems, unusual infections or causes need to be considered. An overgrowth of fungi, usually *Aspergillus* species, can form a ball in the sinuses, usually the maxillary sinus. This will look like a mass filling the sinus on scanning. Polyps look like swellings coming from the lining of the sinus on a CT scan. Allergic polyps commonly occur in the ethmoid sinuses. Angiofibromas are rare and usually cause some distortion of the sinus on a CT scan; they often cause bleeding. Foreign bodies in the sinuses are rare; they sometimes occur as a result of facial trauma.

16. C ★★   OHCS 10th edn → p. 546

Ventilation tubes, or grommets, are the treatment for glue ear which is commoner in Down's syndrome. Glue ear refers to otitis media with effusion and is the main cause of hearing loss in young children. This boy has evidence of hearing impairment on his audiograms. If left untreated, this may seriously affect his learning and development.

17. C ★★   OHCS 10th edn → pp. 570–1

Post-cricoid tumours in the hypopharynx often cause the sensation of a lump in the throat before they interfere with swallowing. As they grow, they cause local pain. They can also cause referred pain to the ear along the sensory fibres of the vagus nerve. This is an ominous sign. Clinical anaemia also indicates that the tumour is advanced.

18. C ★★   OHCS 10th edn → p. 552

A glomus tumour, or non-chromaffin paraganglioma, is a rare vascular benign tumour that arises from the glomus body (a small collection of paraganglionic tissue). These tumours often occur in the middle ear.

Because of blood flow, the tinnitus is pulsatile. A mass may also be felt in the ear. Glomus tumours can also occur in the carotid body but would not give these symptoms.

19. **B** ★★   OHCS 10th edn → p. 568

The cricoarytenoid joints rotate with the vocal cords, so arthritis here causing stiffness can affect the pitch and tone of the voice. This has been reported in 17–70% of patients with rheumatoid arthritis, and airway obstruction by swelling is a rare, but serious, complication.

20. **B** ★★   OHCS 10th edn → p. 554

This is a description of Ménière's disease, which involves attacks of disabling vertigo with unilateral tinnitus and progressive sensorineural hearing loss. Treatment is symptomatic initially. Anti-emetics, such as cyclizine or prochlorperazine, may help to relieve the symptoms but will not reduce the frequency of attacks. Betahistine may be helpful and can be tried, although trial results are equivocal.

21. **E** ★★   OHCS 10th edn → pp. 540, 546

Fluid in the middle ear causes dampening of the tympanic membrane movement and results in hearing impairment and a flat trace on tympanometry. Serous effusion can occur during the resolution of an acute otitis media, probably due to Eustachian tube dysfunction. It will usually resolve within 3 months. Recurrent infections can lead to a cycle of inflammation and can cause chronic suppurative otitis media.

22. **B** ★★

In this emergency situation, the cricothyroid membrane should be identified in the midline, as it is the safest way to approach the airway prior to a formal tracheostomy. When performing a surgical tracheostomy under anaesthesia, a fenestration would be made into the trachea itself, usually at the level of the second or third ring. A cricoid split procedure is very occasionally performed in neonates, and never in an adult. The thyroid cartilage and thyrohyoid membrane should not be entered, as there may be damage to the vocal cords.

23. **A** ★★   OHCS 10th edn → p. 576

The characteristic appearance of this infection is an enlarging, non-tender, violaceous mass. It does not disappear following antibiotic use. It is rare but should be considered.

24. **D** ★★   OHCS 10th edn → p. 554

The unusual feature here is the intention tremor, which should raise suspicion of a brain lesion. Vertigo caused by central lesions is rare, but features in the history may lead you to suspect these. The other tests assess hearing or assess each labyrinth in turn.

25. E ★★

Voice therapy may be all that is required. Surgical approaches employing sharp dissection or laser should only be used if the nodule is resistant to voice therapy. Hypothyroidism is a cause of hoarseness, but not of nodules. Propranolol is used to treat haemangiomata of the larynx, but not nodules.

Surgical versus non-surgical interventions for vocal cord nodules:

→ http://cochranelibrary-wiley.com/doi/10.1002/14651858.CD001934. pub2/full

26. B ★★★

The orbital abscess would be seen on CT scan, and any bony defect would be seen on the CT scan, but not the MRI scan. A sinus X-ray is very rarely performed and would not show details of abscess formation. An ultrasound probe could not be used for an abscess in this location, as it is medial to the orbit and the probe could not be accommodated in the available anatomical space.

→ Rahbar R, Robson C, Petersen RA, *et al*. Management of orbital subperiosteal abscess in children. *Arch Otolaryngol Head Neck Surg*. 2001;**127**:281–6.

27. C ★★★

Children often choke on small foreign bodies, which may become lodged in the airway. If left, they can cause erosion, obstruction, or infection and collapse. Larger objects tend to get stuck in the larynx and may cause airway obstruction or hoarseness. The majority of foreign bodies get stuck in the bronchus and cause unilateral wheeze and breath sounds, and may cause cough. Without the classic history, these may be missed or mistaken for asthma. Although inspiratory and expiratory chest X-rays may be helpful, very young children cannot cooperate with these and a single chest film may miss the diagnosis. To look for the foreign body, the upper and lower airway must be carefully examined with bronchoscopy.

28. C ★★★ OHCS 10th edn → p. 560

Clear fluid that is positive for glucose on a dipstick test suggests a basal skull fracture and leakage of cerebrospinal fluid (CSF). β-2 transferrin is a protein found only in the CSF and perilymph, so it can be used to confirm CSF rhinorrhoea in a suspected basal skull fracture.

29. A ★★★ OHCS 10th edn → p. 560

This boy has a septal haematoma causing the obstruction. The condition is rare but serious and, if left untreated, can cause septal necrosis and collapse. Treatment involves draining it under general anaesthesia and packing the nose. Septoplasty or rhinoplasty may be needed later after fractures if the nose sets abnormally and causes deviation of the septum and blockage or deformity.

30. D ★★★   OHCS 10th edn → p. 560

Batteries are corrosive and require urgent removal.

31. A ★★★   OHCS 10th edn → p. 576

A tumour of the deep lobe of the parotid will medialize the tonsil, and the uvula will be deviated away from the lesion. The facial nerve palsy suggests malignant infiltration of the nerve which lies between the deep and superficial lobes. A lymphoma of the tonsil can medialize the tonsil but would not develop a facial palsy. A retropharyngeal abscess is unusual in this age group and would always be associated with signs of toxicity and a raised temperature. Similarly, a patient with a quinsy or abscess around the tonsil would be in pain. A glomus tumour could produce lower cranial nerve palsies but would not deviate the uvula, as it tends to present lower in the neck.

32. C ★★★★

Following laryngectomy, the potency of the upper airway is lost, and therefore the ability to phonate is lost. There are a variety of ways to restore speech following laryngectomy, and this is a specialist area managed by speech and language therapists.

→ http://www.cancerresearchuk.org/about-cancer/laryngeal-cancer/living-with/speaking-after-laryngectomy

33. E ★★★★   OHCS 10th edn → p. 562

Ongoing epistaxis despite nasal packing is an emergency, and the nose needs to be examined under anaesthesia. The sphenopalatine artery is a branch of the external carotid artery. It passes through the sphenopalatine foramen into the back of the nose. It is distal, so ligation usually controls bleeding, with few complications. Older techniques involving ligation of the external carotid or maxillary artery have higher complication rates.

Chapter 8

Dermatology

Gemma Simcox

Skin disease has a serious impact on an individual's quality of life. It is well recognized that conditions such as psoriasis may have a similar impact on a patient's quality of life to chronic diseases such as diabetes, hypertension, and depression.

Skin problems account for approximately 20% of all patient consultations in primary care in the UK. It is important that clinicians are able to diagnose common skin diseases such as acne, eczema, psoriasis, and cutaneous malignancies and initiate an appropriate management plan. This requires the ability to take a full history and conduct a complete examination. A complete dermatological examination involves examination of the entire skin, mucous membranes, hair, and nails. The description of cutaneous pathologies should include the location and distribution of lesions. The morphology of a lesion or each component of a generalized eruption should be noted. Other organ systems may also need to be examined.

The questions in this chapter will test your knowledge of the skin problems that are frequently encountered in non-specialist clinical practice. Other more rare skin disorders are also covered, either because they are potentially life-threatening or because they are a sign of systemic disease. The questions are designed to improve your ability to recognize the morphology and distribution of cutaneous physical signs.

Hopefully you will find these questions stimulating and an aid to improving your knowledge of skin disease.

QUESTIONS

1. A 42-year-old man with type 2 diabetes has hyperpigmented skin in his axillae, as shown in Figure 8.1 (see Colour Plate section). Which is the single most likely diagnosis? ★

A Acanthosis nigricans

B Atopic eczema

C Erythrasma

D Seborrhoeic dermatitis

E Tinea corporis

2. A 28-year-old man has had red, scaly patches over his cheeks, as shown in Figure 8.2 (see Colour Plate section), for 2 years. He also has scaling of the skin around his eyebrows. Which is the single most likely diagnosis? ★

A Atopic eczema

B Candidiasis

C Psoriasis

D Seborrhoeic dermatitis

E Tinea faciei

3. A 14-year-old girl has lesions on her fingers, as shown in Figure 8.3 (see Colour Plate section). They have been present for 5 months. Which is the single most likely causative organism? ★

A Adenovirus

B Coxsackie virus

C Herpes simplex virus

D Human papillomavirus

E Molluscum contagiosum virus

4. A 23-year-old woman has a rash affecting her forehead, cheeks, and chin, as shown in Figure 8.4 (see Colour Plate section). Which is the single predominant lesion shown here? ★

A Comedone

B Macule

C Nodule

D Papule

E Pustule

5. A 30-year-old woman has had itchy skin for most of her life. Her face is shown in Figure 8.5 (see Colour Plate section). Which is the single most likely diagnosis? ★

A Acne rosacea

B Atopic eczema

C Impetigo

D Psoriasis

E Seborrhoeic dermatitis

6. A 38-year-old woman with lifelong atopic eczema has noticed that her eczema has been getting worse over the past 7 days. She has been taking flucloxacillin for 4 days, but her condition is worsening, as shown in Figure 8.6 (see Colour Plate section), and is becoming painful. Which single treatment should be given? ★

A Betamethasone valerate ointment

B Emulsifying ointment

C IV aciclovir

D IV benzylpenicillin

E Oral metronidazole

7. A 36-year-old man has had a skin rash, as shown in Figure 8.7 (see Colour Plate section), for 20 years. He noticed his nails have become pitted and his scalp scaly. Which is the single most likely diagnosis? ★

A Atopic eczema

B Lichen planus

C Pityriasis versicolor

D Psoriasis

E Seborrhoeic dermatitis

8. A 40-year-old woman attends her general practice (GP) surgery for a Well Woman check-up. She has multiple skin lesions, as shown in Figure 8.8 (see Colour Plate section), that have been present since she was a child and are slowly increasing in number. Which is the single most likely diagnosis? ★

A Epidermoid cysts

B Ganglions

C Neurofibromatosis

D Tuberous sclerosis

E Viral warts

9. A 56-year-old man presents with a thumb that appears as shown in Figure 8.9 (see Colour Plate section). He jammed the thumb in a door a few months ago. The rest of his skin examination is normal. Which is the single most likely diagnosis? ★

A Haematoma

B Lichen planus

C Malignant melanoma

D Onychomycosis

E Psoriasis

10. A 37-year-old woman has painful swollen distal interphalangeal joints. She has the nail changes shown in Figure 8.10 (see Colour Plate section) and says that her nails have been like this for 10 years. Which is the single most likely diagnosis? ★

A Atopic eczema

B Lichen planus

C Psoriasis

D Systemic lupus erythematosus

E Tinea manuum

11. A 40-year-old woman has had a swollen leg for 6 days, as shown in Figure 8.11 (see Colour Plate section). Her temperature is 38.6°C, and her full blood count shows a neutrophil count of 11×10^9/L. Which is the single most likely diagnosis? ★

A Cellulitis

B Deep vein thrombosis

C Psoriasis

D Tinea corporis

E Venous eczema

12. A 40-year-old man has skin between his toes, as shown in Figure 8.12 (see Colour Plate section). Which is the single most likely diagnosis? ★

A Atopic eczema

B Candidiasis

C Psoriasis

D Tinea pedis

E Viral wart

13. A 5-year-old girl has had blisters on her left thigh, as shown in Figure 8.13 (see Colour Plate section), for 2 days. The condition started with a yellow crusted area 5 days ago, which spread, and then the blisters appeared. The girl is otherwise well. Which is the single most likely diagnosis? ★

A Bullous impetigo

B Bullous pemphigoid

C Chronic bullous disease of childhood

D Insect bites

E Scabies

14. A 35-year-old woman has had a skin problem for a number of years. She had a Caesarean section last year, and her scar is shown in Figure 8.14 (see Colour Plate section). Which is the single best description of the appearance? ★

A Auspitz sign

B Impetiginization

C Keloid scar

D Köebner phenomenon

E Striae

15. A 34-year-old man has a lesion on his leg, as shown in Figure 8.15 (see Colour Plate section). He first noticed it about 2 months ago. Which is the single most likely diagnosis? ★

A Actinic keratosis

B Benign naevus

C Bowen's disease

D Malignant melanoma

E Seborrhoeic keratosis

16. A 10-month-old baby has had skin lesions, as shown in Figure 8.16 (see Colour Plate section), for 2 days. He had an upper respiratory tract infection last week but seems to be well in himself now. The lesions appear to be in a different place from the ones he had yesterday. Which is the single most likely diagnosis? ★

A Acute urticaria

B Atopic eczema

C Erythema multiforme

D Meningococcal septicaemia

E Urticaria pigmentosa

17. A 28-year-old woman developed a rash on her body 1 week ago. Today it has spread to her hands, as shown in Figure 8.17 (see Colour Plate section). Three weeks ago, she had a 3-day course of trimethoprim to treat a urinary tract infection. Which is the single most likely diagnosis? ★

A Acute urticaria

B Allergic contact eczema

C Erythema multiforme

D Erythema nodosum

E Psoriasis

18. A 64-year-old man has had a sore back and mouth for 2 months. These are shown in Figure 8.18 (a, b) (see Colour Plate section). Which is the single most likely diagnosis? ★

A Bullous pemphigoid

B Erythema multiforme

C Herpes simplex virus infection

D Lichen planus

E Pemphigus vulgaris

19. A 30-year-old man with ulcerative colitis has lesions on his anterior shins. The lesions started to develop 7 months ago and are getting bigger. They are shown in Figure 8.19 (see Colour Plate section). Which is the single most likely diagnosis? ★

A Erythema nodosum

B Leukocytoclastic vasculitis

C Necrobiosis lipoidica

D Pyoderma gangrenosum

E Venous ulcers

20. A 60-year-old man has a lesion on his arm that has grown rapidly over the past 3 weeks and that is not painful. It is shown in Figure 8.20 (see Colour Plate section). Which is the single most likely diagnosis? ★

A Actinic keratosis

B Basal cell carcinoma

C Keratoacanthoma

D Malignant melanoma

E Seborrhoeic keratosis

21. A 22-year-old man has a lesion on his lower abdomen that is increasing in size and which is shown in Figure 8.21 (see Colour Plate section). He has tried 1% hydrocortisone cream, to no avail. Which is the single most appropriate treatment? ★

A Betamethasone valerate cream

B Ketoconazole shampoo

C Oral flucloxacillin

D Oral prednisolone

E Oral terbinafine

22. A 45-year-old man had a cardiac transplant 8 years ago. He has developed a painful lesion on his forehead that is irregular in shape with a thick crust. The lesion has grown rapidly over the past 3 months. Which is the single most likely diagnosis? ★

A Actinic keratosis

B Bowen's disease

C Malignant melanoma

D Seborrhoeic keratosis

E Squamous cell carcinoma

23. An 18-year-old man has severe scarring acne with multiple nodules and cysts on his face, which has been getting progressively worse over the past 5 years. Treatment with oxytetracycline for 8 months has not helped. He is otherwise well. Which is the single most appropriate treatment? ★

A 5% benzoyl peroxide cream

B Clobetasone butyrate cream

C Oral erythromycin

D Oral isotretinoin

E Oral prednisolone

24. A 3-month-old baby has a rash on his groin. He is otherwise well. The rash is shown in Figure 8.22 (see Colour Plate section). Which is the single most appropriate treatment to prescribe? ★

A 1% hydrocortisone cream

B Aqueous cream

C Fucidin cream

D No treatment

E Nystatin cream

25. A 56-year-old woman has a sore, red, dry, itchy rash that is confined to her face. It has developed over the past month. The rest of her skin is normal. She is otherwise well and is taking no medication. Which is the single most likely diagnosis? ★

A Acne rosacea

B Allergic contact dermatitis

C Atopic eczema

D Seborrhoeic dermatitis

E Systemic lupus erythematosus

26. The nose of a 69-year-old man has the appearance shown in Figure 8.23 (see Colour Plate section). It has looked like this for 9 years. Which is the single best term to describe the appearance? ★ ★

A Acne vulgaris

B Lupus pernio

C Lupus vulgaris

D Rhinophyma

E Wegener's granulomatosis

27. A 26-year-old man with atopic eczema has lesions on his palms, as shown in Figure 8.24 (see Colour Plate section), which are very itchy. They come and go, and seem to flare up when the rest of his eczema is bad. He has not yet tried any treatments, as he is unsure which of them to use. Which is the single most appropriate treatment? ★ ★

A 1% hydrocortisone ointment

B 5% permethrin cream

C Aciclovir cream

D Betamethasone valerate ointment

E Ketoconazole cream

28. A 12-year-old boy has had atopic eczema for many years. He is concerned about paler patches on his face, shown in Figure 8.25 (see Colour Plate section), which have been present for the past 6 months. He has changes consistent with eczema over the rest of his skin, but no pigmentary change. Which is the single most likely diagnosis? ★ ★

A Cutaneous T-cell lymphoma

B Pityriasis alba

C Seborrhoeic dermatitis

D Tinea faciei

E Vitiligo

29. A 78-year-old woman has an itchy rash over her trunk and limbs, as shown in Figure 8.26 (see Colour Plate section). She has been itchy for several weeks, and blisters appeared last week. She is not taking any regular medication. Which is the single most likely diagnosis? ★★

A Bullous pemphigoid

B Erythema multiforme

C Pemphigus vulgaris

D Psoriasis

E Scabies

30. A 47-year-old man has had a rash over both lower legs for 2 days, as shown in Figure 8.27 (see Colour Plate section). He was treated with amoxicillin for a throat infection last week. Which is the single most likely diagnosis? ★★

A Cellulitis

B Erythema multiforme

C Erythema nodosum

D Leukocytoclastic vasculitis

E Streptococcal septicaemia

31. A 36-year-old woman is concerned about the pigmentation on her cheeks, shown in Figure 8.28 (see Colour Plate section), which is spreading. She is not taking any medication. Which is the single most appropriate treatment? ★★

A Betamethasone valerate cream

B High-factor sunblock

C Hydroquinone cream

D Hydroxychloroquine

E Oral prednisolone for 6 weeks

32. A 30-year-old woman gave birth 7 weeks ago. She has had a lesion on her breast for 2 weeks. It bleeds profusely and interferes with breastfeeding of her baby. Which is the single most likely diagnosis? ★★

A Bacillary angiomatosis

B Granuloma annulare

C Pyoderma gangrenosum

D Pyogenic granuloma

E Viral wart

33. A 30-year-old man has been on a walking holiday in Spain and now has blisters, shown in Figure 8.29 (see Colour Plate section). The remainder of his skin is normal. Which is the single most likely diagnosis? ★★

A Allergic contact eczema

B Bullous pemphigoid

C Impetigo

D Insect bite reaction

E Linear immunoglobulin A (IgA) disease

34. A 38-year-old man with coeliac disease has a very itchy rash over his buttocks and a similar rash over the elbows and knees, shown in Figure 8.30 (see Colour Plate section). Which is the single most likely diagnosis? ★★

A Atopic eczema

B Dermatitis herpetiformis

C Lichen planus

D Psoriasis

E Scabies

35. An 18-month-old girl has a widespread rash on her trunk. It started to develop 2 weeks ago with a single round red plaque, 2 cm in diameter, on her left flank. This was treated with a topical antifungal cream, with no effect. During the last 3 days, several more scaly plaques have appeared over the trunk. These are 1 cm in diameter and pink in the centre, with a dark red ring around the outside. They are itchy. The girl is well in herself and is thriving. Which is the single most likely diagnosis? ★★★

A Guttate psoriasis

B Pityriasis rosea

C Seborrhoeic dermatitis

D Tinea corporis

E Viral exanthema

36. A 63-year-old man is referred for treatment of the lesion shown in Figure 8.31 (see Colour Plate section). Which single treatment modality should be offered? ★★★

A Cryotherapy

B Direct excision and primary closure

C Mohs micrographic surgery

D Radiotherapy

E Topical 5-fluorouracil (5FU)

37. A 55-year-old woman has a patch of hair loss over the parietal region of the scalp, as well as an atrophic lesion over her ear, as shown in Figure 8.32 (see Colour Plate section). Which is the single most likely diagnosis? ★★★★

A Alopecia areata

B Discoid lupus

C Lichen planopilaris

D Psoriasis

E Tinea capitis

ANSWERS

1. A ★   OHCS 10th edn → p. 588

This condition is commoner in patients with type 2 diabetes and obesity. It causes velvety, hyperpigmented plaques in the axillae, groin, and neck folds. It can be associated with other underlying causes such as polycystic ovaries, Cushing's syndrome, and acromegaly and can also be drug-induced. As such, it is advised to take a full history from the patient. Acanthosis nigricans itself is harmless; weight loss and treatment of any underlying conditions *may* improve the appearance of the lesions. There is an association with internal malignancy (mostly gastrointestinal); however, this is very rare and the onset of symptoms is usually more rapid.

→ http://www.nhs.uk/conditions/acanthosis-nigricans/Pages/Introduction.aspx

2. D ★   OHCS 10th edn → p. 596

This common dermatosis causes scaling and erythema in the nasolabial folds, eyebrows, and hairline. There may be associated fine scale on the scalp and within the ears. This distribution rather than in the flexures (eczema), extensors (psoriasis) or an asymmetrical distribution is typical of tinea or candida, both of which favour warm, moist sites. Seborrhoeic dermatitis is often associated with yeast infections and, as such, treatment is aimed to target this, as well as the eczematous inflammatory response, with emollients and mild topical steroids. The treatments will need to be specific to the area affected, e.g. shampoo for scalp.

→ https://cks.nice.org.uk/seborrhoeic-dermatitis

3. D ★   OHCS 10th edn → p. 599

These are viral warts, caused by human papillomavirus. This is a very common presentation in general practice and, in most cases, requires no treatment but can cause pain and distress. There are several options for therapy, including topical cytotoxic agents, cryotherapy, and duct tape, all of which require perseverance. Fifty per cent of warts resolve within 6 months without treatment.

→ http://patient.info/doctor/viral-warts-excluding-verrucae

→ http://www.nhs.uk/Conditions/Warts/Pages/Introduction.aspx

4. E ★   OHCS 10th edn → p. 585

A comedone can be open (blackhead) or closed (whitehead). A macule is a flat, distinct lesion/area of skin, up to 1 cm in diameter (plaque greater than 1 cm). A nodule is a solid, palpable lesion, up to 10 mm in diameter. A papule is a solid, palpable lesion, up to 5 mm in diameter. A pustule is a papule or nodule containing purulent material.

5. B ★   OHCS 10th edn → p. 596

Atopic eczema is classically itchy and typically affects flexural sites. It is common for there to be facial involvement, as seen here.

Acne rosacea would not be expected to be itchy. Impetigo again would not itch and would be of a short duration, rather than lifelong. Impetigo may affect a patient with eczema, as the skin barrier is not as effective. However, the picture would note well-defined patches of yellow, crusting plaques or blistering which are not seen here. The final two conditions given as options are psoriasis and seborrhoeic dermatitis. Psoriasis is also not itchy (although it can be sore at times), and the latter tends to be confined to the nasolabial folds and eyebrows, which are not noted in the illustration.

→ http://www.dermnetnz.org/topics/atopic-eczema/

→ http://www.eczema.org/basic-treatment

6. C ★   OHCS 10th edn → p. 599

This is eczema herpeticum (eczema infected with herpes simplex virus). Note the characteristic monomorphic vesicles. The history of the eczema getting worse despite antibiotic treatment is a clue. This infection spreads very quickly and requires IV treatment. The patient will present feeling unwell with a fever and the characteristic rash, as illustrated in Figure 8.6 (although initially there may be fewer vesicles). This is a dermatological emergency and requires admission and often IV antiviral treatment.

→ https://www.nice.org.uk/guidance/qs44/chapter/quality-statement-7-treatment-of-eczema-herpeticum

7. D ★   OHCS 10th edn → p. 594

Note the symmetrical distribution of plaques with a silvery scale on the surface. The extensor aspects of the elbows are involved—a classic site for psoriasis. The additional information of the nails and scalp gives the final clue of psoriasis and should always form part of the examination of the dermatology patient. Lichen planus (LP) can affect the nails, from dystrophy to total nail destruction, which is different from pitting. LP can, in addition, also affect the scalp with a form of scarring alopecia, which is quite different from the thick scale of scalp psoriasis. LP and psoriasis both koebnerize, but LP classically affects the volar aspect of the wrist and can also affect mucosal surfaces. Pityriasis versicolor causes altered skin pigmentation secondary to a yeast infection, rather than thickened plaques. Atopic eczema and seborrhoeic dermatitis have been noted in previous questions.

→ https://www.nice.org.uk/guidance/cg153

→ http://patient.info/doctor/chronic-plaque-psoriasis

8. C ★

This is neurofibromatosis type 1. It is an autosomal dominant condition. The multiple dome-shaped tumours are neurofibromas. There may also be café-au-lait macules and axillary freckling of the skin. Epidermoid cysts tend to occur in isolation, certainly not in the numbers shown in the illustration. Ganglions are also solitary and should be found on the limbs. The skin manifestation of tuberous sclerosis are numerous and include café-au-lait spots, shagreen patches, and skin tags.

→ http://www.nfauk.org (Neurofibromatosis Association)

→ http://www.tuberous-sclerosis.org/about-tsc.html

9. C ★   OHCS 10th edn → p. 592

This is an acral subungual melanoma. Note the pigmentation of the skin around the nail (Hutchinson's sign). The nail has been distorted by the growth of the melanoma under the nail bed. As noted in previous questions, psoriasis causes nail pitting; lichen planus causes nail dystrophy and destruction. Fungal nail infection is known as onychomycosis and requires nail clippings for laboratory analysis prior to treatment.

→ http://www.dermnetnz.org/topics/nail-terminology/

→ http://www.pcds.org.uk/clinical-guidance/nails

10. C ★   OHCS 10th edn → p. 594

The severe nail dystrophy, swollen distal interphalangeal joints, and fine scaling over the fingertips are suggestive of psoriasis. Approximately 5% of patients with psoriasis develop arthropathy. Joint involvement would not be expected with atopic eczema or tinea manuum (the history is also a little too prolonged for tinea). The nail changes associated with lichen planus have been noted previously. Systemic lupus erythematosus does have dermatological sequelae, in particular discoid lupus erythematosus which mainly affects the scalp and sun-bearing areas. There can be nail changes, but those tend to be limited.

→ http://www.jabfm.org/content/22/2/206.full

→ http://www.dermnetnz.org/topics/discoid-lupus-erythematosus/

11. A ★

A patient with a hot, red, swollen leg may have cellulitis or deep vein thrombosis. In this case, the raised temperature, the sharp demarcation of the erythema at the ankle, and the neutrophilia support the diagnosis of cellulitis. A common cause for cellulitis and recurrent cellulitis is tinea pedis, and this should be treated to prevent recurrence. Treatment should include the commonest pathogens, i.e. streptococci and *Staphylococcus*.

→ http://bestpractice.bmj.com/best-practice/monograph/63.html

12. D ★   OHCS 10th edn → p. 598

This is 'athlete's foot'. Note the macerated and scaled appearance of the skin in the web space.

13. A ★   OHCS 10th edn → p. 598

Impetigo can cause tense blisters, as shown here. Note the yellow, crusted patches, which are more typical of impetigo seen in children. Bullous pemphigoid would not be seen at this age, and scabies would present with a more widespread, intensely pruritic rash. The lesions may have started as simple insect bites which have become secondarily infected.

→ http://patient.info/doctor/impetigo-pro

14. D ★   OHCS 10th edn → p. 584

The Köebner phenomenon describes the occurrence of skin lesions in areas of trauma or surgery. It occurs with psoriasis (as seen here), warts, vitiligo, and lichen planus.

The Auspitz sign is small areas of bleeding when removing scale from plaques, which may indicate psoriasis. Impetiginization merely describes a lesion that has become secondarily infected. Striae are stretch marks, and a keloid scar is a specific type of scarring characterized by raised, red scar.

→ http://www.dermnetnz.org/topics/the-koebner-phenomenon/

15. D ★   OHCS 10th edn → p. 592

Note the irregular colour of, and edge to, this lesion. Remember the ABCDE for pigmented lesions:

- asymmetry
- border
- colour
- diameter >7 mm
- evolution.

There is a movement towards a 7-point checklist for the identification of a suspected malignant melanoma. However, the ABCDE rules are helpful to use with patient self-monitoring. Lesions scoring 3 or more should be referred. This is based on major features scoring 2 each and minor features scoring 1. A lesion that stands out from the others is always cause for concern.

→ https://cks.nice.org.uk/melanoma-and-pigmented-lesions#!diagnosissub

16. A ★   OHCS 10th edn → p. 603

These are wheals. The history of them being present for less than 24 hours is typical. Acute urticaria can result from infection, drugs, or a food allergy, but often no cause is found. The lesions of erythema multiforme are targetoid, and these lesions are also not typical of meningococcal septicaemia, which has palpable, dark purple plaques. Urticaria pigmentosa tends to have a more prolonged course and the lesions are lighter brown.

→ http://patient.info/doctor/urticaria-pro

17. C ★   OHCS 10th edn → p. 588

The targetoid lesions are typical of erythema multiforme. This usually starts on the trunk and spreads acrally (to the hands, feet, and head). Common causes are drugs and infection (typically herpes simplex virus or *Mycoplasma* infection). Lesions of erythema nodosum would usually be found on the anterior shins and without the typical targetoid pattern.

→ http://www.dermnetnz.org/topics/erythema-multiforme/

→ http://www.pcds.org.uk/clinical-guidance/erythema-nodosum

18. E ★   OHCS 10th edn → p. 602

Note the eroded areas from superficial blisters that have burst. This is typical of pemphigus vulgaris. The skin around the eroded areas is normal (in contrast, in bullous pemphigoid, it is erythematous). The erosions on the lip further support the diagnosis of pemphigus vulgaris.

→ http://www.pemphigus.org.uk

19. D ★   OHCS 10th edn → p. 588

This condition is commoner in patients with inflammatory bowel disease. Note the ulcers with a purple-red border. The ulcers often appear undermined at the edge. Surgical intervention will make this condition worse and may lead to limb amputation, so do not cut these lesions out! Treatment options include topical, intralesional, and oral steroids and biological therapy. Erythema nodosum presents as subcutaneous nodules; these lesions are not vasculitic in nature which would exclude answer B. They can often mistakenly be treated as venous ulcers over some time, but attention must be given to the site (not in the gaiter area), age of the patient, and the characteristics of the lesions themselves. Necrobiosis lipoidica are distinct yellow/brown patches on the shins.

→ http://www.pcds.org.uk/clinical-guidance/pyoderma-gangrenosum

→ http://www.dermnetnz.org/topics/necrobiosis-lipoidica/

20. C ★   OHCS 10th edn → p. 590

This nodule is growing rapidly and has a symmetrical dome shape with a central plug of keratin. These lesions are usually excised in order to differentiate them from a squamous cell carcinoma. This is very typical of this type of lesion.

→ http://patient.info/doctor/keratoacanthoma-pro

21. E ★   OHCS 10th edn → p. 598

This is tinea corporis (incognito). It has been exacerbated by the topical steroid that this patient has used. An oral antifungal agent is needed. Once a topical steroid has been used on tinea corporis/pedis/manuum, the symptoms will reduce, but the rash itself will spread (tinea incognito). Oral antifungal agents are indicated. This can be the case for some time and, as such, it is important to take a thorough history of the start of the symptoms.

→ http://www.dermnetnz.org/topics/tinea-incognito/

22. E ★   OHCS 10th edn → p. 590

This describes an exophytic tumour with a hyperkeratotic crust on a sun-exposed site. Squamous cell carcinoma is commoner in organ transplant recipients as a result of immunosuppressive medication, so it must always be considered.

→ https://www.dermnetnz.org/topics/squamous-cell-carcinoma-of-the-skin

23. D ★   OHCS 10th edn → p. 600

For severe acne, isotretinoin for 16 weeks is the drug of choice. However, close supervision is required, as it has significant side-effects. Up to 80% of patients have side-effects and the potential list is long. Significant ones to note are depression, dry lips and skin, effects on the liver and lipids, and an association with birth defects. Oral and topical steroids should be avoided in acne.

→ https://cks.nice.org.uk/acne-vulgaris

24. E ★   OHCS 10th edn → p. 598

The satellite pustules that are visible are characteristic of candidiasis. The folds are involved (which makes an extrinsic dermatitis, such as irritant dermatitis, unlikely). This infection is treated with an antifungal cream such as nystatin. Aqueous cream should be avoided, as it can itself cause irritation.

→ http://www.dermnetnz.org/topics/candida/

25. B ★   OHCS 10th edn → p. 596

The distribution of this eruption gives the clue that this is allergic contact eczema—the eczema is limited to one body site. The face is a common site to be affected by allergic contact dermatitis (common allergens are make-up and hair dye). As noted in previous questions, seborrhoeic dermatitis does not tend to be itchy, nor does rosacea. The cutaneous manifestations of systemic lupus erythematosus can affect the face and are classically described as a malar rash (butterfly distribution) over the cheeks, with a sore mouth and sun sensitivity.

→ http://www.pcds.org.uk/clinical-guidance/eczema-contact-allergic-dermatitis-including-latex-and-rubber-allergy

26. D ★★   OHCS 10th edn → p. 600

This bulbous swelling of the nose has occurred as a result of long-standing rosacea. The tissues have been infiltrated by granulomatous inflammation. This is very distinctive. Lupus pernio is cutaneous sarcoid and is characterized by bluish red nodules over the nose. Lupus vulgaris is cutaneous tuberculosis and again has a very distinctive appearance.

→ http://patient.info/doctor/rosacea-and-rhinophyma

27. D ★★

This is pompholyx hand eczema. It consists of very itchy vesicles and papules on the palms. Scabies is less likely in this patient, because the papules come and go together with the rest of his eczema. This form of eczema requires treatment with a potent topical corticosteroid such as betamethasone valerate. There is no evidence of an infection—an infection, whether viral, bacterial, or fungal, would tend to produce an asymmetrical rash or an asymmetrical exacerbation of an existing inflammatory dermatoses.

→ http://www.dermnetnz.org/topics/pompholyx/

28. B ★★   OHCS 10th edn → p. 586

The patches here have an indistinct border and are hypopigmented (not sharp-edged and depigmented, as would be seen in vitiligo). This is pityriasis alba, which occurs on the faces of children with atopic eczema. It improves with treatment with emollients and mild topical corticosteroid creams. Seborrhoeic dermatitis may cause changes in skin pigmentation, but this is far less common. Tinea faciei is a fungal infection on the face and presents in the same manner as on the body/feet. This would be a very unusual age for cutaneous T-cell lymphoma.

→ http://www.dermnetnz.org/topics/pityriasis-alba

29. A ★★   OHCS 10th edn → p. 602

Note the tense blisters on an erythematous urticated base. Bullous pemphigoid does not usually affect the mucosal membranes. The lesions in the illustration are very typical for this condition.

→ http://www.dermnetnz.org/topics/bullous-pemphigoid/

30. D ★★   OHCS 10th edn → p. 588

This is a small-vessel vasculitis causing palpable purpura of the skin. This was the result of a hypersensitivity reaction to amoxicillin. Whenever purpura is seen, it is important to think of systemic sepsis. However, this man is well and has too long a history for this to be the diagnosis.

→ http://www.dermnetnz.org/topics/leukocytoclastic-vasculitis-pathology/

31. B ★★

This is melasma. The safest treatment is to advise the daily use of a sunblock. Sunshine makes this condition worse. Some women develop melasma while pregnant or when taking the oral contraceptive pill. Hydroquinone can be damaging to the skin, especially at high strength.

→ http://patient.info/doctor/melasma-chloasma-pro

32. D ★★   OHCS 10th edn → p. 602

This is a benign vascular tumour that is commoner in pregnancy. Lesions are often triggered by trauma. They can be easily removed with minor surgery or cryotherapy for smaller lesions. Some may resolve spontaneously. Granuloma annulare is a distinctive annular collection of smooth papules.

→ http://www.dermnetnz.org/topics/pyogenic-granuloma/

33. D ★★

Note the tense blisters in this case. The surrounding skin is normal, which makes bullous pemphigoid, linear IgA disease, and allergic contact eczema unlikely. There is no evidence of impetigo here. Linear IgA disease can present in childhood and adulthood with grouped lesions and, as noted earlier, the surrounding skin is often affected. IgA autoantibodies are directed against the basement membrane.

→ http://patient.info/doctor/linear-iga-dermatosis

34. B ★★

The key is the relationship to coeliac disease. This can be considered a dermatological manifestation of the disease and is treated with strict adherence to a gluten-free diet plus dapsone.

→ http://www.dermatitisherpetiformis.org.uk

35. B ★★★   OHCS 10th edn → p. 586

This is a fairly typical description of pityriasis rosea. The condition starts with a herald patch, which is the key to diagnosis. This is a round plaque, 1–2 cm in diameter, with a pink centre separated from a dark red edge by a fine, scaly area. One to two weeks later, a secondary rash appears, which is usually on the trunk in a symmetrical distribution. These lesions look like smaller versions of the herald patch, and the rash is usually itchy. Guttate psoriasis is very unusual in young children and tends to form drop-like salmon-pink lesions with a fine scale. Seborrhoeic dermatitis causes dry, flaky skin, often on the scalp, but it can occur in folds and flexural areas. Tinea is a fungal infection, and it usually responds to antifungal agents. A single red, inflamed patch tends to keep growing, with the outer edge more inflamed like a ring. Viral exanthemata are typically erythematous maculopapular rashes that occur with a viral upper respiratory infection.

→ http://www.dermnetnz.org/topics/pityriasis-rosea/

36. C ★★★

Mohs micrographic surgery is now routinely offered to patients with basal cell carcinoma (BCC), as in this case, and squamous cell carcinoma (SCC) on high-risk sites on the face where it is important to preserve as much healthy tissue as possible. Direct excision and closure would not be the preferred option at this site, due to unknown margins and also poor cosmetic result. Cryotherapy, topical therapy such as 5FU, or radiotherapy would not be appropriate, as it would not expect to achieve either a tissue diagnosis or a curative resection, although they do all have roles in the treatment of skin malignancy.

→ https://www.nice.org.uk/guidance/csg8

37. B ★★★★   OHCS 10th edn → p. 589

The diagnosis can be very difficult if the symptoms are confined only to the scalp, but in this case, there is the addition of atrophic lesions in the ears which is typical of discoid lupus. Lichen planopilaris would typically present with frontal loss of hair and scarring alopecia; however, the skin may look slightly scaly or merely scarred, with few visible hair follicles. Alopecia areata is a non-scarring form of hair loss. Psoriatic patients have very thick, adherent scale, particularly around the nape of the neck.

→ http://www.dermnetnz.org/topics/discoid-lupus-erythematosus/

Chapter 9

Anaesthesia and intensive care

Alex Bonner

Anaesthesia is a relatively young specialty by comparison with its counterparts. William Morton administered the first anaesthetic in 1846 in Boston, Massachusetts, and the Royal College of Anaesthetists was cleaved from the Royal College of Surgeons in 1948. Now anaesthetists form the largest group of hospital-based doctors.

Anaesthetists are highly trained physicians whose role is by no means limited to the operating theatre. They oversee the patient journey through the peri-operative period, i.e. preoperative assessment and optimization of the sick surgical patient, ensuring safe intra-operative provision of anaesthesia as well as care of the patient in the early postoperative period. Anaesthetic skills are also requested during management of the critically ill in the Emergency Department, during the care of the parturient mother in providing analgesic, anaesthetic, and intensive care input, and increasingly in the pre-hospital environment. Anaesthetists have an important role in the practice of intensive care where complementary experience in medicine is useful. Other roles of the anaesthetist include provision of acute and chronic pain services. and subspecialty interests include regional, paediatric, cardiothoracic, vascular, and neuroanaesthesia.

Anaesthesia is a highly practical specialty, with a strong emphasis on the basic sciences underpinning its practice. Physiology and pharmacology exert their effects with immediacy; therefore, an affinity for these disciplines is desirable. Anaesthetists need to be able to assimilate knowledge of the basic sciences with skills in history and examination, in order to plan for, and respond to, patient needs. In answering these questions, you will be asked to use similar skills.

QUESTIONS

1. A 70-year-old man has had worsening shortness of breath for 2 days. He has a 50-pack-year history of cigarette smoking but otherwise has no previous medical history. He appears unwell, with a reduced level of consciousness and inadequate respiratory effort. The following arterial blood gas levels are obtained while he is breathing through a face mask with a reservoir bag, with an oxygen flow rate of 15 L/minute:

- pH 7.14
- pO_2 10.1 kPa
- pCO_2 9.8 kPa
- bicarbonate 29.2 mmol/L
- base excess +9.4.

Which is the single best description of the acid–base derangement? ★

A Metabolic acidosis with respiratory compensation

B Metabolic alkalosis with respiratory compensation

C Mixed respiratory and metabolic acidosis

D Respiratory acidosis with evidence of metabolic compensation

E Respiratory acidosis with no evidence of metabolic compensation

2. A 19-year-old man fractured his right lower leg about 30 minutes ago while playing football. He was carried off the pitch on a stretcher. He is in pain and there is some bloodstaining on his sock. His right lower leg is immobilized in a box splint. He has an open fracture of his right distal tibia. There is no distal neurovascular deficit and he is haemodynamically stable; blood loss is estimated to be minimal. He has no other injuries and is fully alert. Which is the single most appropriate initial analgesia to administer? ★

A Intramuscular (IM) diclofenac

B Intravenous (IV) alfentanil

C IV morphine

D IV paracetamol

E Oral codeine phosphate

3. A 19-year-old woman is brought into the Emergency Department by paramedics. She was found unconscious in her bed by her parents who found empty packets of several prescription medications and a bottle of vodka. She does not open her eyes at all but withdraws to pain. She makes no verbal response. Which single number reflects her Glasgow Coma Scale score? ★

A 3

B 6

C 9

D 12

E 15

4. A 56-year-old man underwent primary percutaneous coronary intervention (PCI) for an anterior myocardial infarction 6 hours ago. His pain had eased, but he suddenly had severe central crushing chest pain radiating into his left arm. He is now unconscious, with no signs of life. The defibrillator is attached, and the monitor displays the rhythm shown in Figure 9.1 (see Colour Plate section). Cardiopulmonary resuscitation (CPR) with chest compressions and bag–valve–mask ventilation is started. He has intravenous (IV) access. Which is the single next most appropriate management? ★

A Continue CPR for 2 minutes

B Defibrillation

C Endotracheal intubation

D IV atropine

E IV adrenaline (epinephrine)

5. A 24-year-old woman is about to undergo a surgical procedure under a nerve block. Shortly after the anaesthetist finishes the procedure, she feels light-headed and dizzy. She experiences ringing in her ears and tingling around her mouth. Which is the single most likely diagnosis? ★

A Acute labyrinthitis

B Anaphylaxis

C Failure of anaesthetic

D Local anaesthetic toxicity

E Vasovagal attack

6. A 34-year-old woman has been admitted to hospital with cellulitis of her forearm. She has just been given her second dose of intravenous (IV) flucloxacillin. She now has chest tightness and difficulty in breathing, and feels dizzy. She has a diffuse urticarial rash all over her body, and bilateral expiratory and inspiratory wheeze. Her pulse rate is 120 bpm, her blood pressure 80/40 mmHg, and her oxygen saturation 91% on room air. Which is the single most appropriate initial management? ★

A Intramuscular (IM) adrenaline (epinephrine) 0.5 mg

B IV chlorphenamine 10 mg

C IV adrenaline (epinephrine) 1 mg

D IV hydrocortisone 100 mg

E Take blood for serum mast cell tryptase

7. A 76-year-old woman had a left total knee replacement 4 days ago. She is normally fit and healthy. She has had an uncomplicated post-operative recovery, but recent observations give her a Modified Early Warning Score (MEWS) of 6, whereas 1 hour ago, the score was 2. Her pulse rate is 120 bpm, her blood pressure 90/45 mmHg, her oxygen saturation 90% on room air, her respiratory rate 30 breaths/minute, and her temperature 37.5°C. She is alert but has chest pain and shortness of breath. Which is the single most likely cause of her acute deterioration? ★

A Cardiac tamponade

B Myocardial infarction

C Pneumonia

D Pneumothorax

E Pulmonary embolism

8. A 19-year-old man has had a recurrent dislocation of his left shoulder. He has been given 20 mg of intravenous (IV) midazolam and his shoulder is now reduced. He is now unconscious and has stopped breathing. Which is the single most appropriate immediate management? ★

A Connect electrocardiographic (ECG) monitoring

B Give IV flumazenil

C Give IV naloxone

D Intubate the patient

E Open the airway with a jaw thrust

9. A 63-year-old woman had a redo total hip replacement under general anaesthesia 3 days ago. She now has chest pain which developed suddenly and is worse on inspiration. Her pulse rate is 110 bpm, her oxygen saturation 90% on 5 L of oxygen by mask, and her temperature 37.4°C. Which single investigation is likely to confirm the diagnosis? ★

A Chest X-ray

B Computed tomography (CT) pulmonary angiogram

C Electrocardiogram (ECG)

D Echocardiography

E Cardiac enzymes

10. A 64-year-old woman had an inferior myocardial infarction (MI) 12 hours ago and has been successfully revascularized. She suddenly develops a profound narrow complex bradycardia with a rate of 30 bpm. Her blood pressure is 75/39 mmHg, and she feels dizzy and sick. Which is the single most appropriate immediate management? ★

A Intravenous (IV) amiodarone

B IV atropine

C IV isoprenaline

D Transcutaneous (external) cardiac pacing

E Transvenous cardiac pacing

11. A 6-week-old boy, who was born prematurely, has had vomiting and lethargy for 5 days. He has sunken eyes and reduced skin turgor. His capillary refill time is 4 seconds. The following arterial blood gas sample is obtained:

- pH 7.52
- P_aCO_2 5.0 kPa
- P_aO_2 11.0 kPa
- HCO_3 34.2 mmol/L
- base excess +9.1.

Which is the single best description of his metabolic status? ★

A Metabolic acidosis without respiratory compensation

B Metabolic alkalosis with respiratory compensation

C Metabolic alkalosis without respiratory compensation

D Respiratory alkalosis with metabolic compensation

E Respiratory alkalosis without metabolic compensation

12. A 68-year-old man has chronic obstructive pulmonary disease (COPD). He has been involved in a motor vehicle collision and has a fractured femur and signs of a tension pneumothorax. His oxygen saturation is 76% on room air. He is being prepared for a needle thoracocentesis. Which is the single most appropriate means of oxygen delivery to use? ★

A Face mask continuous positive airway pressure (CPAP)

B Immediate intubation and ventilation

C Nasal cannulae

D Non-rebreather mask with reservoir bag

E Venturi mask with 35% oxygen delivery

13. A 55-year-old woman with a history of chronic pain presents to the Emergency Department with morning somnolence, blurred vision, and urinary retention. She states that her general practitioner has recently started a new chronic pain medication, but she cannot remember the name of the drug. Which single drug, used in the treatment of chronic pain, is most likely to cause this group of side-effects? ★ ★

A Amitriptyline

B Carbamazepine

C Gabapentin

D Morphine

E Sodium valproate

14. A 35-year-old man is seen on the day-case unit prior to an arthroscopy for knee pain. He describes himself as 'fit and well' and does not smoke. He takes inhalers for asthma, which is well controlled, and has no other medical problems. Which single American Society of Anesthesiologists (ASA) grade best describes his physical status? ★ ★

A I

B II

C III

D IV

E V

15. A 31-year-old woman is scheduled for an elective laparoscopic cholecystectomy. After intubation, the CO_2 (capnography) trace diminishes; she begins to desaturate, and the anaesthetist is unable to hear air entry when auscultating over the chest despite being able to hand-ventilate her easily. Which is the single most likely cause for this? ★★

A Anaphylaxis

B Cardiac arrest

C Monitoring failure

D Oesophageal intubation

E Bilateral pneumothoraces

16. Urgent help is required in the anaesthetic room. A patient has suddenly become unwell during induction of anaesthesia. He has generalized muscle rigidity and tachycardia, and appears sweaty. His blood pressure is normal. Which is the single most likely diagnosis? ★★

A Acute dystonia

B Anaphylaxis

C Epileptic seizure

D Malignant hyperthermia

E Suxamethonium apnoea

17. A 49-year-old woman has presumed sepsis arising from her biliary tract. She is known to have hypertension and gallstones. The admitting team have obtained intravenous (IV) access and taken blood. The woman has also received a dose of broad-spectrum antibiotics. Her blood pressure is 91/40 mmHg and her serum lactate level is 3.6 mmol/L. Which is the single most important next management step, according to the Surviving Sepsis Campaign? ★★

A Commence a vasopressor infusion

B Give a minimum 20 mL/kg fluid bolus

C Insert a peripheral arterial line

D Insert a central venous catheter

E Recheck the serum lactate level

18. A new mother on the obstetric ward had a forceps delivery under epidural anaesthesia 2 days ago. She initially made a good recovery and was walking on the ward. However, she now has back pain, leg weakness, and bladder dysfunction. She has lower limb motor and sensory dysfunction on testing. Which is the single most likely diagnosis? ★★

A Bacterial meningitis

B Brown-Séquard syndrome

C Epidural haematoma

D Peroneal nerve palsy

E Prolapsed intervertebral disc

19. A previously fit and well 34-year-old man is undergoing surgery for a fractured right femur. He is under a general anaesthetic and the orthopaedic surgeons have just inserted the femoral nail. Intra-operative blood loss is estimated to be about 2000 mL. He has been given 3000 mL of intravenous (IV) crystalloid fluid throughout the operation. A bedside haemoglobin test reads 6.9 g/dL. His pulse rate is 100 bpm and his blood pressure is 125/75 mmHg. No further blood loss is anticipated. Which is the single most appropriate next step in management? ★★

A Administration of recombinant activated factor VIIa

B Prescribing post-operative iron tablets

C Transfusion of fully cross-matched blood

D Transfusion of group O rhesus-negative blood

E Transfusion of group-specific blood

20. A 53-year-old woman is transferred to the recovery room after a laparoscopic cholecystectomy. The procedure was technically difficult and lasted longer than anticipated. Her temperature in recovery is 32.9°C. Which single physical process accounts for the greatest heat loss intra-operatively? ★★

A Conduction

B Convection

C Humidification

D Radiation

E Respiration

21. A 31-year-old man has sustained a laceration to his right (dominant) hand while at work. The laceration is on the palm of the hand on the radial aspect. A median nerve block at the wrist is planned to provide sufficient anaesthesia for the wound to be explored and sutured. Which single option most accurately describes where the median nerve lies at the wrist? ★ ★

A Between the tendons of the palmaris longus and the flexor pollicis longus

B Lateral to the radial artery

C Medial to the ulnar artery

D Medial to the ulnar nerve

E Superficial to the flexor retinaculum

22. A 17-year-old man has HbAS (sickle cell trait). He is undergoing repair of a fractured radius under general anaesthesia. During the procedure, the surgeon uses a tourniquet to create a bloodless field, and K-wires the fracture. The patient receives intravenous (IV) fluid and analgesia, and post-operatively is given oxygen. Which single factor is associated with an increased risk of sickle cell crisis in this case? ★ ★

A IV fluid therapy

B Opioid analgesia

C Oxygen therapy

D Prophylactic antibiotics

E Tourniquet use

23. An 82-year-old man has had a transurethral resection of the prostate (TURP) procedure under spinal anaesthetic. The procedure was long and the surgeon required large volumes of irrigating fluid. In recovery, the patient becomes increasingly agitated and confused; his Glasgow Coma Scale score falls and he requires intubation. Which is the single most likely metabolic abnormality to account for this? ★ ★

A Hyperglycaemia

B Hypernatraemia

C Hypoglycaemia

D Hypokalaemia

E Hyponatraemia

24. A 24-year-old woman is 32 weeks pregnant with her first child. She has had pregnancy-induced hypertension. Her booking blood pressure was 125/76 mmHg. She has come to the labour suite with a headache and she has some ankle oedema. Her blood pressure is now 145/92 mmHg, and urinalysis shows 3+ proteinuria. She suddenly loses consciousness and has a tonic–clonic seizure. She is put in the recovery position and given supplementary oxygen. Which is the single most appropriate treatment? ★ ★ ★

A Intravenous (IV) lorazepam

B IV magnesium sulfate

C IV phenytoin

D Oral methyldopa

E Sublingual nifedipine

25. A 20-year-old man is undergoing his first ever general anaesthetic for an elective tonsillectomy. Shortly after administration of the induction agents, he becomes unwell. Which is the single most likely first sign indicating that he may be having an anaphylactic reaction? ★ ★ ★

A Angio-oedema

B Cough

C Desaturation

D Hypotension

E Rash

26. A 6-year-old child weighing approximately 20 kg is brought into the Emergency Department. She has sustained burns to the torso, covering an estimated 20% of body surface area (BSA). The child is haemodynamically stable. Which is the single correct volume of fluid to administer in the first 8 hours following admission? ★ ★ ★

A 250 mL

B 400 mL

C 600 mL

D 800 mL

E 1000 mL

27. A 42-year-old woman had a partial thyroidectomy 24 hours ago. Her preoperative haemoglobin level was 11.4 g/dL. Today's result is 3.8 g/dL. She is pain-free; her pulse rate is 85 bpm, and her blood pressure is 118/76 mmHg. Blood loss was estimated to be about 300 mL, and there is minimal fluid in the surgical drain. Her neck is not distended, and the wound site is clean and dry. Which is the single most likely cause of the anaemia? ★ ★ ★

A Bone marrow failure

B Iron deficiency

C Major intra-operative haemorrhage

D Ongoing post-operative haemorrhage

E Spurious result

28. A 29-year-old man has been on the Intensive Therapy Unit for 2 days following a serious motor vehicle collision. He is making no respiratory effort, and tests confirm brainstem death. The medical team is planning to talk to the relatives about the possibility of organ donation. Which single advice is correct in relation to organ donation? ★ ★ ★ ★

A Organs can only be harvested once the donor's heart has stopped beating

B Organ donation can only take place if the donor is on the organ donor register or carried an organ donation card

C Organs of patients who are human immunodeficiency virus (HIV)-positive are usually taken

D Organs will usually be harvested if the donor is on the organ donation register, even if the next of kin do not wish for organs to be donated

E The next of kin can specify if they do not want particular organs to be donated

29. A 35-year-old woman is undergoing a diagnostic laparoscopy for pelvic pain. She is deemed to be at high risk for post-operative nausea and vomiting. Which single class of drugs can be used in the prophylaxis of post-operative nausea and vomiting? ★ ★ ★ ★

A Anticonvulsants

B Benzodiazepines

C Corticosteroids

D Opioids

E Smooth muscle relaxants

30. An 80-year-old woman is undergoing palliative care for inoperable cancer. She has copious secretions in the upper airway that are troublesome, and is requesting something to relieve this symptom. Which single group of drugs is the most appropriate to prescribe? ★★★★

A Acetylcholinesterase inhibitors
B Anticholinergic agents
C Antihistamines
D Dopamine antagonists
E Sympathomimetic agents

ANSWERS

1. D ★

The blood gas shows a marked respiratory acidosis. As is common in patients with smoking-related lung disease, a degree of metabolic compensation for a chronically elevated pCO_2 occurs, shown by the raised bicarbonate level. However, this man is unwell with a grossly elevated pCO_2, which exceeds the buffering capacity of the blood. He has a reduced level of consciousness from carbon dioxide narcosis.

Table 9.1 sets out a step-by-step guide on how to approach blood gases:

Table 9.1 Flow chart

Acidosis: pH 7.35	Alkalosis: pH 7.45
Look at the base excess first. Normal (−3 to +3) = respiratory acidosis, and pCO_2 will be raised (>6 kPa)	Look at the base excess first. Normal (−3 to +3) = respiratory alkalosis, and pCO_2 will be low (<4.5 kPa)
High negative (> −4) = metabolic acidosis. If pCO_2 is normal (4.5–6 kPa), it is just a metabolic acidosis. If pCO_2 is low (<4.5 kPa), there is respiratory compensation. If the pCO_2 is also high, it is a mixed acidosis	High positive (> +4) = metabolic alkalosis. If pCO_2 is normal (4.5–6 kPa), it is just a metabolic alkalosis. If pCO_2 is high (>6 kPa), there is respiratory compensation. If pCO_2 is low, it is a mixed alkalosis
High positive (> +4) = respiratory acidosis with renal compensation. The pCO_2 will be high (>6 kPa)	High negative (> −4) = respiratory alkalosis with renal compensation. The pCO_2 will be low (<4.5 kPa)

2. C ★   OHCS 10th edn → p. 636

Acute severe pain is best managed with strong opioids such as morphine. Common routes of administration include the IV, IM, oral, intranasal, and subcutaneous routes. IV administration will provide the most rapid pain relief and avoids first-pass metabolism by the liver (first-pass metabolism mainly affects orally administered drugs). The strong opioids should be titrated to effect. The IM route is useful in a ward setting, but perfusion to peripheral muscles can be impaired due to the sympathetic activity that follows acute injury. This results in delayed onset of action, with potentially late onset of side-effects once perfusion to muscle is restored, and would be less suitable in this setting. Alfentanil is a very short-acting opioid that is usually only used in the operating theatre or given by infusion for its sedative effect.

The World Health Organization (WHO) analgesic ladder offers a step-wise approach to pain management, although the severity of acute pain needs to be assessed to ensure that treatment begins on the appropriate 'rung' of the ladder.

Treatment of this patient with paracetamol or a weak opioid alone would be insufficient to control his acute pain. Combining a strong opioid with paracetamol and a non-steroidal anti-inflammatory drug (e.g. diclofenac or ibuprofen) will reduce the overall amount of opioid that is needed to control his pain. This is beneficial, as it will minimize the risk of opioid side-effects (sedation, nausea and vomiting, constipation, etc.).

→ http://www.ganfyd.org/images/thumb/7/77/WHO_Analgesic_Ladder. png/550px-WHO_Analgesic_Ladder.png

3. B ★   OHCS 10th edn → p. 778

The Glasgow Coma Scale (GCS) is used to assess and record the level of consciousness of a patient. Although it was developed for use on traumatized patients, the GCS is used to assess virtually all patients who present with a depressed level of consciousness, irrespective of the cause. See Table 9.2.

Table 9.2 Glasgow Coma Scale

Best eye response	Score
No eye opening	1
Eyes open to pain	2
Eyes open to command	3
Eyes open spontaneously	4
Best motor response	
No motor response	1
Extensor posturing to pain	2
Abnormal flexor posturing to pain	3
Withdraws to pain (normal flexion)	4
Localizing response to pain	5
Obeys command	6
Best verbal response	
No sounds	1
Incomprehensible sound	2
Inappropriate speech	3
Confused conversation	4
Normal	5

Reprinted from *The Lancet*, 304, Teasdale G, Jennett B, Assessment of coma and impaired consciousness: A Practical Scale, pp. 81–84, Copyright (1974) with permission from Elsevier.

4. B ★

This man has ventricular fibrillation (VF) and requires immediate electrical defibrillation. The fibrillating heart has electrical activity, but this is uncoordinated and so the heart cannot function as a pump. Passing electricity through the heart (defibrillation) causes transient cessation of all endogenous electrical activity. Once this occurs, the intrinsic pacemakers should take over and result in coordinated contractions of the atria and ventricles being resumed.

Chest compressions alone are very unlikely to cardiovert VF into a per-fusing rhythm, and if a defibrillator is immediately available, a defibrillating shock should be given as soon as VF is identified. Once VF has been identified, the initial shock takes precedence over airway, breathing, and the administration of any drugs.

The stepwise management of VF and pulseless ventricular tachycardia (VT) are the same and are outlined in the adult Advanced Life Support algorithm.

→ https://www.resus.org.uk/resuscitation-guidelines/

5. D ★   OHCS 10th edn → p. 632

Whenever local anaesthetic is used, the possibility of toxicity should be considered. The first symptoms of local anaesthetic toxicity are due to central nervous system (CNS) stimulation (tinnitus, circumoral paraesthesiae, light-headedness, and dizziness), followed by CNS depression and cardiovascular collapse. Injection of local anaesthetic should always follow careful aspiration to ensure that the needle is not in a blood vessel. If a patient complains of symptoms suggestive of toxicity, the operator should immediately stop injecting the anaesthetic. The management of local anaesthetic toxicity can be aided by the administration of Intralipid®.

→ http://www.aagbi.org/sites/default/files/la_toxicity_2010_0.pdf

6. A ★

This patient is having an anaphylactic reaction, probably to the administered antibiotics. The priorities in management should follow the Airway, Breathing, Circulation approach (see the adult Advanced Life Support algorithm).

If anaphylaxis is suspected, the precipitant should be stopped (e.g. stop antibiotic infusion) and the patient given IM adrenaline 0.5 mg (0.5 mL of 1:1000 adrenaline). It is unlikely that IM adrenaline will cause an adverse event if it later transpires that the patient was not having an anaphylactic reaction. If in doubt, IM adrenaline should be given.

Chlorphenamine, hydrocortisone, and taking blood for mast cell tryptase are all indicated in cases of anaphylaxis, but adrenaline takes priority. Common precipitants of anaphylaxis include blood products, colloid fluids, antibiotics, and muscle relaxants.

→ http://www.resus.org.uk/pages/anaalgo.pdf

7. E ★

This woman has had lower limb surgery and is likely to have been fairly immobile for the last 4 days. She is at high risk of a deep vein thrombosis and subsequent pulmonary embolism. This is the most likely pathology.

Beck's triad (muffled heart sounds, raised jugular venous pressure, and hypotension) would make cardiac tamponade more likely, but this is not pathognomonic. Equally, there is no history of ischaemic heart disease, and an acute myocardial infarction is unlikely to give rise to desaturation unless there has been gross heart failure. Pneumonia is relatively common in the post-operative population but usually has a more gradual onset of cough, pyrexia, anorexia, and lethargy. Pneumothoraces can be rapid in onset, but again there is no reason (e.g. pre-existing lung disease, positive pressure ventilation, central lines, etc.) to suggest that this patient is at risk from these.

The MEWS is an objective way of highlighting adverse patient physiology, so that appropriate help can be sought (see Table 9.3).

Table 9.3 Modified Early Warning Score (MEWS)

Total score	Action
2	Repeat observations in 30 minutes
3	Inform a junior doctor
>4	Request a junior doctor immediately

Source data from QJM: An International Journal of Medicine, 94, 10, Subbe CP, Kruger M, Validation of a modified Early Warning Score in medical admissions, pp. 521–526, 2001, Oxford University Press.

The MEWS is calculated as shown in Table 9.4.

Table 9.4 MEWS calculation

	3	2	1	0	1	2	3
Respiratory rate (breaths/minute)		<9		9–14	15–20	21–29	≥30
Heart rate (bpm)		<40	41–50	51–100	101–110	111–129	≥130
Systolic blood pressure (mmHg)	<70	71–80	81–100	101–199		≥200	
Temperature (°C)		<35		35–38.4		≥38.5	
AVPU				Alert	Reacts to Voice	Reacts to Pain	Unresponsive

Reproduced from QJM: An International Journal of Medicine, 94, 10, Subbe CP, Kruger M, Validation of a modified Early Warning Score in medical admissions, pp. 521–526. Copyright © 2001, Oxford University Press.

8. E ★

This patient has respiratory depression secondary to benzodiazepine excess. The immediate approach to any critically ill patient begins with airway assessment and management if indicated. This must take place before moving on to breathing and then to circulation, as outlined in the adult Advanced Life Support (ALS) algorithm. If the patient's airway is not patent or safe after a jaw thrust and use of airway adjuncts (e.g. Guedel airway), they may need intubation. Applying ECG leads is part of the assessment of the circulation.

Naloxone is the reversal agent used in opioid overdose. Flumazenil is the reversal agent used in benzodiazepine overdose, but again airway management takes precedence over flumazenil in this case.

→ http://www.resus.org.uk/pages/als.pdf

9. B ★

This history points towards the diagnosis of pulmonary embolism in the post-operative period. Pelvic surgery and orthopaedic surgery are risk factors for pulmonary embolism. Although a chest X-ray and an ECG may point towards pulmonary embolism, in most hospitals, the 'gold standard' investigation for confirming the diagnosis is CT pulmonary angiography.

10. B ★

This patient has a bradycardia, which is probably secondary to her inferior MI and which is causing cardiovascular compromise (hypotension). In accordance with the Adult Bradycardia Algorithm, she has adverse signs of her bradycardia, and the first-line treatment should be with IV atropine (an anticholinergic drug). If the bradycardia persists, IV isoprenaline (a β-adrenoceptor agonist) and transcutaneous (external) and temporary cardiac pacing may all be utilized.

Amiodarone is used to treat tachyarrhythmias and often results in bradycardia.

→ https://www.resus.org.uk/resuscitation-guidelines/

11. C ★ OHCS 10th edn → p. 172

A child with pyloric stenosis classically presents with a metabolic alkalosis due to loss of acid from the upper gastrointestinal tract. A flow chart giving a step-by-step guide on how to approach blood gases is shown in Answer 1.

12. D ★

This man's tension pneumothorax is life-threatening. He also needs a high concentration of oxygen to be delivered to his functioning lung, as he is grossly hypoxaemic. Some colleagues may voice concern that a patient with COPD potentially has a 'hypoxic drive' and that giving oxygen will cause the patient to hypoventilate, retain carbon dioxide, and become drowsy. This is not a concern in this life-threatening emergency setting—the patient is likely to die of hypoxaemia or circulatory collapse secondary to the tension pneumothorax first, unless he is treated. The oxygen concentration can be reduced once the patient is more stable.

A face mask with a non-rebreather valve and reservoir bag will deliver about 80% oxygen when the oxygen is turned on to 15 L/minute. Nasal cannulae will deliver about 28%, and the Venturi system will deliver 35%, both of which are insufficient in this setting. Face mask CPAP is likely to expand this pneumothorax further, as would intubation and ventilation. A chest drain must be sited before commencing either of these in this situation.

13. A ★★

Amitriptyline is a tricyclic antidepressant, but it is also used in the treatment of neuropathic pain. This class of drugs has an analgesic effect that is independent of any antidepressant effect. The drug blocks many neurotransmitters in the central nervous system, including noradrenaline and serotonin, but it is the anticholinergic actions that would cause the side-effects described here. Drugs that antagonize acetylcholine at cholinergic receptors (e.g. atropine and hyoscine) often cause these effects.

The other drugs are all used in the treatment of chronic pain. All of these agents have significant side-effects. Titrating drugs to achieve the right balance between the desired effect and tolerable side-effects is paramount in this setting. Warning patients about what side-effects to expect and how to manage them is an important aspect of drug prescribing. For example, morning somnolence (tiredness) may be overcome by taking the evening dose 1 or 2 hours earlier.

14. B ★★   OHCS 10th edn → p. 615

Class II refers to a patient with a mild systemic disease. The ASA grading of patient status was introduced in the 1960s. Although simple, it has been shown to correlate with the risks associated with anaesthesia and surgery, and therefore forms part of the preoperative assessment of all patients undergoing general anaesthesia. See Table 9.5.

Table 9.5 ASA grading

ASA grade	Description	Mortality rate (%)
I	A normal healthy patient	0.1
II	A patient with mild systemic disease	0.2
III	A patient with severe systemic disease	1.8
IV	A patient with severe systemic disease that is a constant threat to life	7.8
V	A moribund patient who is not expected to survive without the operation	9.4
VI	A declared brain-dead patient whose organs are being removed for donor purposes	

The mortality rates quoted above are an average for both elective and emergency surgery. The suffix E is added to denote an emergency operation.

15. D ★★ OHCS 10th edn → p. 627

Anaphylaxis usually presents with a combination of bronchospasm, rash, tachycardia, and hypotension. As the patient is easy to hand-ventilate, anaphylaxis is unlikely, as bronchospastic lungs require high airway pressures.

Cardiac arrest would cause an absent pulse oximetry trace, and breath sounds would still be audible while the patient was being hand-ventilated.

A failure of monitoring equipment is unlikely to give this picture, as both the capnography and the pulse oximetry modules would have to be faulty at the same time, and the patient might well become cyanotic.

The occurrence of bilateral pneumothoraces would be very unlucky but could give rise to this situation. However, probability dictates that this is very unlikely.

Oesophageal intubation is the most likely cause here and could be confirmed by auscultating over the stomach and hearing air entry when hand-ventilating the patient. Its management involves removal of the misplaced tube, re-oxygenating the patient with mask ventilation, and then intubating the trachea.

16. D ★★ OHCS 10th edn → p. 628

Malignant hyperthermia is an inherited disorder of calcium metabolism that affects skeletal muscle. It is most often triggered by suxamethonium or the volatile anaesthetic agents. Its presentation varies from one individual to another, but it should be considered when there is unexplained tachycardia, especially in the presence of tachypnoea, muscle rigidity, or an increase in end-tidal pCO_2. Malignant hyperthermia can be a life-threatening condition, or it may present more insidiously. Emergency management includes removal of the trigger agent, cooling, and treatment with dantrolene (a drug that interferes with skeletal muscle contraction). Without treatment, the mortality rate is approximately 75%; with treatment, mortality is significantly reduced.

None of the other diagnoses classically present as described here. Acute dystonia is often triggered by neuroleptic agents and typically presents in the first few days of new treatment. It is rarely associated with anaesthesia. Suxamethonium apnoea is an inherited deficiency of plasma cholinesterase, resulting in delayed metabolism of suxamethonium and therefore prolongation of neuromuscular blockade.

17. B ★★

Vasoactive mediators from the infective agent and from damaged endothelium are causing widespread vasodilatation, hypotension, and a resultant tachycardia. The first goal of the management of septic shock is to ensure adequate filling (pre-load), as measured by the central venous pressure (CVP). Once the patient is adequately filled, if hypotension and shock persist, a vasopressor should then be commenced, such as noradrenaline (norepinephrine) which acts predominantly upon α_1-adrenoceptors.

A central line will allow the CVP to be measured, but more important than the specific value recorded is the trend in pressure in response to fluid boluses. If the CVP continues to rise, this usually suggests that more fluid is needed, whereas a plateau in the CVP suggests that adequate filling has been achieved. A central line will also allow some drugs to be administered that would otherwise be irritant to smaller peripheral veins.

An arterial line will be useful in the High-Dependency Unit/Intensive Therapy Unit setting but is not a priority in the first instance. Similarly, rechecking the serum lactate level is unlikely to be of use within the first 6 hours.

18. C ★★

The history points to a rare, but very serious, complication of epidural anaesthesia. A haematoma that is formed following insertion of a catheter into the epidural space can expand and cause neurological compromise. Traumatic insertion or derangements of clotting increase the likelihood of haematoma formation.

19. C ★★

Loss of more than 20% of the circulating volume is regarded as a significant blood loss, and in most circumstances, this needs to be replaced with a blood transfusion. Circulating volume is approximately 70 mL/kg, so it is around 4900 mL in a 70-kg man. In this case, there is time to obtain fully cross-matched blood, which usually takes up to 45 minutes to become available. This blood will be thoroughly matched for the patient's blood group (A, B, AB, or O), rhesus D status (negative or positive), and the rarer antibodies/antigens. Type-specific blood takes about 20 minutes to become available and is matched for blood group and rhesus D status, but not for the rarer antibodies/antigens. Group O rhesus-negative blood (universal donor blood) should be available immediately in most clinical areas but carries the risk of the patient raising antibodies to the rarer antigens, which can cause problems with future blood transfusions. The decision as to which blood to request will depend upon the level of clinical urgency.

The following link is to the National Blood Service website.

→ https://www.blood.co.uk

20. D ★★

Radiation accounts for approximately 40% of the heat lost from the body. In addition, convection (30%), respiration (including humidification) (20%), and conduction (10%) are all important, and their relative contributions vary, depending on the environment. Space blankets are designed to reduce heat loss from radiation.

21. A ★★ OHCS 10th edn → p. 749

The median nerve lies between the two prominent tendons at the wrist (the palmaris longus and flexor pollicis longus) and is deep to the flexor retinaculum within the carpal tunnel. Swelling within the carpal tunnel gives rise to 'carpal tunnel syndrome', which is caused by compression upon the median nerve.

The ulna bone, ulnar nerve, and ulnar artery are medial to the median nerve, and the radial artery lies lateral to it.

22. E ★★

Use of a tourniquet is associated with precipitation of sickle cell crisis. If a tourniquet must be used, the limb should be thoroughly exsanguinated prior to inflation. All of the other options are associated with minimization of the risk of a crisis and should form part of the peri-operative care where appropriate.

23. E ★★

TURP syndrome is a complication of TURP and is caused by the combination of fluid overload and hyponatraemia, which results from high volumes of hypotonic irrigating fluid being used over the open prostate gland. It can be complicated by hyperglycinaemia (not hyperglycaemia) as a result of the glycine irrigation fluid that is used by the surgeons. Therefore, the mental state of these patients should be regularly assessed peri-operatively, and any sign of confusion should be a cause for concern. Long procedures are a risk factor for TURP syndrome. Management consists of slow correction of the underlying metabolic disturbance. Rapid correction of hyponatraemia can cause permanent neurological disability.

24. B ★★★ OHCS 10th edn → p. 49

This patient initially had pre-eclampsia. This condition is diagnosed after 20 weeks' gestation when there is hypertension (systolic blood pressure greater than 140 mmHg and/or diastolic blood pressure greater than 90 mmHg) or a rise in systolic blood pressure of more than 30 mmHg or a rise in diastolic blood pressure of more than 15 mmHg, compared with the booking blood pressure, and greater than 300 mg/dL per 24 hours of protein in the urine (in practical terms, more than 2+ on urinalysis). Eclampsia is diagnosed when a patient with pre-eclampsia has a seizure. The Magpie Trial demonstrated that patients with pre-eclampsia were less likely to go on to develop eclampsia if they were given IV magnesium. This and other work has also formed the basis of the first-line treatment of eclampsia with IV magnesium.

→ The Magpie Trial Collaborative Group. Do women with preeclampsia, and their babies, benefit from magnesium sulphate? The Magpie Trial: a randomised placebo-controlled trial. *Lancet*. 2002;**360**:1331–2.

→ http://emedicine.medscape.com/article/261435-overview

25. D ★★★   OHCS 10th edn → p. 237

Hypotension is observed more commonly than any other clinical sign in patients who are developing anaphylactic reactions. Any of the other signs mentioned may still occur.

→ http://www.aagbi.org/safety/allergies-and-anaphylaxis

26. D ★★★   OHCS 10e → p. 766

Approximately 50 000 children present to Emergency Departments with burns every year in the UK. Estimation of the area affected is an important part of the initial assessment and is aided by the use of a Lund–Browder chart. Although fluid resuscitation in burns has been controversial, the Parkland formula is widely used in the management of paediatric burns. The take-home message is that fluid requirements are high because of losses through the damaged skin barrier.

Parkland formula: for the first 24 hours after the burn, give 4 mL/kg per % BSA burn of Hartmann's solution. Give half of this volume in the first 8 hours after the burn, and the other half in the next 16 hours.

27. E ★★★

There is no suggestion that there was significant intra-operative or post-operative bleeding, so major blood loss is unlikely. Iron deficiency anaemia is a chronic pathology and would take longer than 24 hours to develop. Bone marrow failure can result in anaemia but is relatively rare and usually causes a pancytopenia, so it would be important to check the platelet and white cell counts too. Most importantly, this patient has no features of profound anaemia such as circulatory collapse (shock).

The most likely cause is a spurious result due to either an error when taking the blood sample (e.g. taking it from the drip arm and causing dilution) or a laboratory error (this is much less likely). As there are no features of circulatory compromise, a new sample should be taken and analysed. Spurious laboratory results are not uncommon, and if you ever doubt the clinical likelihood of a result, you should consider repeating the investigation.

28. E ★★★★

The majority of organ donations in the UK occur from heart-beating donors. The use of non-heart-beating donors is increasing in the UK but is still relatively uncommon. A patient does not have to be registered on the organ donor register to donate organs, but if they expressed the view that they would not want to donate organs during life, this decision is usually honoured. If a patient expressed the view that they wanted to donate their organs, but their living next of kin were against organ donation, it is unlikely that organs would be taken.

→ http://www.organdonation.nhs.uk

29. C ★★★★

Dexamethasone (a corticosteroid) is commonly used as an anti-emetic. It is usually given intra-operatively, as it is associated with unpleasant side-effects when given to patients who are awake.

30. B ★★★★

Anticholinergic drugs (e.g. hyoscine) are routinely used for their antisialagogue effect, particularly in the palliative care setting. Acetylcholine is the neurotransmitter at muscarinic receptors of the parasympathetic nervous system, responsible for control of secretions. Therefore, anticholinergic drugs will block this pathway.

Chapter 10

Eponymous syndromes

Luci Etheridge and Alex Bonner

Eponyms are still widely used in medicine. Most commonly, they describe collections of clinical features (i.e. a syndrome) or particular clinical signs but are also used to name procedures, anatomy, and equipment. As our understanding of pathophysiology and genomics has improved, naming of diseases and clinical signs has tended to reflect that. However, many eponyms still persist from an era when naming patterns of disease or illness presentation enabled clinicians to gather data, recognize problems, and decide on treatments before the pathology or treatment was fully understood. In this chapter, you will be asked questions challenging your ability to recognize clinically relevant eponyms that you may well encounter in your practice as a doctor.

QUESTIONS

1. A 16-year-old girl is referred to the gynaecology clinic as she has never menstruated. She is 140 cm tall. She has small breast bud development and sparse pubic and axillary hair present. Inspection of the external genitalia is normal. A trans-abdominal ultrasound scan shows her ovaries and uterus to be present, but are small and physiologically quiescent. Her initial blood tests are as follows:

- follicle-stimulating hormone (FSH) 60 IU
- luteinizing hormone (LH) 48 IU
- prolactin 410 IU.

What is the single most likely diagnosis? ★

A Congenital paramesonephric duct obstruction

B Hypothalamic hypogonadism

C Mayer–Kuster–Hauser–Rokitansky syndrome

D McCune–Albright syndrome

E Turner's syndrome

2. A 6-hour-old term baby boy weighs 2.54 kg. He has microcephaly, a flat occiput, upward-slanting palpebral fissures, a protruding tongue, a single palmar crease on the right hand but normal palmar creasing on the left, and a wide sandal gap. Which is the single most likely finding on neurological examination? ★ ★

A Absent Moro reflex

B Exaggerated Moro reflex

C Generalized hypertonia

D Generalized hypotonia

E Selective hypertonia of the lower limbs

3. A 68-year-old man with a history of alcohol abuse presents with an acute abdomen. He has a 12-hour history of back pain. On examination, Grey Turner's sign is present. Which is the single most likely pathophysiological process to account for this? ★ ★

A Obstructive jaundice

B Pleural effusion

C Polycythaemia

D Retroperitoneal haemorrhage

E Ureteric colic

4. A previously fit and well 50-year-old man has a left-sided facial weakness, which he first noticed that morning. There is no history of any associated pain or rash. On examination, he has a lower motor neurone weakness, power 0/5 on the left side of his face, and he is unable to fully close his left eye. Examination is otherwise normal, and his blood pressure is 132/84 mmHg. Which is the single best next course of action? ★★

A Admit to hospital for an urgent head computed tomography (CT) scan

B Prescribe 20 mg prednisolone for 14 days

C Prescribe 60 mg prednisolone for 5 days

D Prescribe 60 mg prednisolone with 800 mg aciclovir for 5 days

E Refer urgently to ear, nose, and throat (ENT)

5. A 57-year-old man has had worsening pain in his left shoulder blade for 2 weeks which is keeping him awake at night. It is now spreading along the medial side of his left arm, and he has numbness and tingling in the little finger of his left hand. On examination, he has reduced power in the fourth and fifth fingers on the left, drooping of his left eyelid, and constriction of the left pupil. What is the single most important investigation to confirm the likely diagnosis? ★★

A Bone scan

B Chest X-ray

C Computed tomography (CT) scan thorax

D Magnetic resonance imaging (MRI) scan brain and neck

E Nerve conduction studies

6. You are asked to perform an arterial blood gas sample on a 20-year-old man who has been admitted to hospital with pneumonia. In preparation, you perform Allen's test. Which is the single most likely anatomical explanation of a positive test? ★★★

A Impaired digital blood flow

B Incomplete palmar arch

C Raynaud's disease

D Subclavian vein thrombosis

E Thoracic outlet obstruction

7. A 53-year-old man has sudden-onset leg weakness and altered sensation. A magnetic resonance imaging (MRI) spine has revealed a lesion consistent with a partial Brown-Séquard syndrome. Which single answer best describes the signs expected on clinical examination? ★ ★ ★

A A spastic paralysis on the contralateral side of the body below the level of the lesion, with contralateral loss of fine touch sensation, vibration touch, and proprioception, and ipsilateral loss of pain and temperature sensation

B A spastic paralysis on the contralateral side of the body below the level of the lesion, with contralateral loss of pain and temperature sensation and ipsilateral loss of fine touch sensation, vibration touch, and proprioception.

C A spastic paralysis on the same side of the body below the level of the lesion, with ipsilateral loss of fine touch sensation, vibration, proprioception, pain, and temperature

D A spastic paralysis on the same side of the body below the level of the lesion, with ipsilateral loss of fine touch sensation, vibration, and proprioception, and contralateral loss of pain and temperature sensation

E A spastic paralysis on the same side of the body below the level of the lesion, with ipsilateral loss of pain and temperature sensation, and contralateral loss of fine touch sensation, vibration, and proprioception

8. A patient is admitted to the Medical Admissions Unit with a provisional diagnosis of Ludwig's angina. What is the single most likely anatomical site of the presenting problem? ★ ★ ★

A Anterior neck

B Central chest

C Floor of mouth

D Left arm

E Mandible

9. A 10-month-old boy is admitted to hospital with a chest infection. He has always had difficulty feeding, but this seems to have worsened and he coughs and splutters with his feeds and often sounds 'chesty'. He has faltering growth, having dropped from the 75th centile at birth to the 9th centile now. He has developmental delay and is not yet rolling and is unable to sit. On examination, he has lots of upper airway sounds apparent. He has a flat, broad nasal bridge, a prominent forehead, and a prominent tongue. He has contractures of his wrists and elbows, with truncal hypotonia. He has marked hepatosplenomegaly. What single finding would you expect on analysis of his urine? ★ ★ ★ ★

A Altered organic acid pattern

B Excess glycosaminoglycans

C Generalized aminoaciduria

D Microscopic haematuria

E Presence of reducing substances

10. A 10-year-old boy has a small, deformed right-sided chest wall. His right middle and ring finger are fused together. A computed tomography (CT) scan shows absence of his right pectoralis major muscle. What is the single most likely diagnosis? ★ ★ ★ ★

A Down's syndrome

B Muscular dystrophy

C Pectus carinatum

D Pectus excavatum

E Poland syndrome

11. A 75-year-old woman with a history of rheumatic fever presents with worsening breathlessness and features of acute heart failure. On examination, you notice that her head is nodding in synchrony with the heart beat—De Musset's sign. Which is the single most likely valvular lesion to account for this? ★ ★ ★ ★

A Aortic regurgitation

B Aortic stenosis

C Mitral stenosis

D Mitral regurgitation

E Pulmonary stenosis

12. A 76-year-old man presents to the Emergency Department with a chronically discharging left ear and pain behind his left eye. His temperature is 38.5°C. On examination, he has a sixth cranial nerve palsy on the left side. Which is the single most likely syndrome to explain these findings? ★ ★ ★ ★

A Ganser syndrome

B Gilbert's syndrome

C Goldenhar syndrome

D Gradenigo's syndrome

E Guillain–Barré syndrome

13. A 45-year-old man is involved in a motorcycle accident. He presents to the Emergency Department, complaining of pain in his right forearm. X-rays demonstrate a Galeazzi fracture. Which is the single best description of the abnormalities seen on the X-ray? ★ ★ ★ ★

A A dorsally angulated fracture of the distal radius

B A fracture of both the mid-shaft radius and ulna

C A fracture of the proximal ulna with a dislocation of the radial head

D A fracture of the radius with an associated dislocation of the distal radio-ulnar joint

E An intra-articular fracture of the distal radius

ANSWERS

1. E ★   OHCS 10th edn → pp. 250, 655

Turner's syndrome is a common cause of primary amenorrhoea and should be considered in all girls presenting with this. It is caused by a chromosome abnormality, with a karyotype of 45,XO. Girls are typically short and, if left untreated, will only grow to less than 5 feet on average. They have typical features, which include webbing of the neck, lymphoedema, a low posterior hairline, wide-spaced nipples, and a wide carrying angle. Ovaries do not develop properly, causing post-menopausal levels of gonadotrophin hormones and affecting the development of secondary sexual characteristics. In hypothalamic hypogonadism, the levels of follicle-stimulating hormone (FSH) and luteinizing hormone (LH) are low. Congenital paramesonephric duct obstruction is an example of a congenital Müllerian duct abnormality, which causes anatomical abnormalities of the uterus and ovaries, as is Mayer–Kuster–Hauser–Rokitansky syndrome. McCune–Albright syndrome affects bones and endocrine tissues and causes precocious puberty, rather than delayed puberty. If left untreated, this can also cause short stature.

2. D ★★   OHCS 10th edn → pp. 152–3

These are the classic phenotypic features of a baby with trisomy 21 (Down's syndrome). The consistent neurological finding in babies with trisomy 21 is generalized hypotonia—they are floppy babies.

3. D ★★★

Grey Turner's sign describes bruising present on the flanks of a patient following retroperitoneal haemorrhage. It is often described in association with acute pancreatitis, but there are other causes of retroperitoneal haemorrhage. Cullen's sign is peri-umbilical discoloration, and Fox's sign describes discoloration of the inguinal crease, both caused by haemorrhage tracking along tissues planes.

4. C ★★   OHCS 10th edn → p. 575

This man has Bell's palsy (Charles Bell). This is treated with a course of high-dose prednisolone; it is not recommended to treat with antiviral treatment. There is no history of a rash that would suggest Ramsay Hunt syndrome, which is treated with aciclovir. Diagnosis is a clinical one, so no investigations are needed. The majority of cases resolve within 9 months. Urgent referral should be done if there is any doubt about the diagnosis, or in recurrent or bilateral Bell's palsy. Routine referral should be considered if there is no improvement clinically within 1 month.

→ https://cks.nice.org.uk/bells-palsy

5. **C** ★★   OHCS 10th edn → p.424

The description on examination is of an ulnar nerve palsy—paraesthesiae and weakness in the fourth and fifth fingers—and Horner's syndrome (Johann Friedrich Horner, Swiss ophthalmologist, 1869)—ipsilateral ptosis and miosis. The third part of the triad in Horner's syndrome is anhidrosis, loss of facial sweating, but this is often not reported and harder to find on examination. The story of severe shoulder pain, in combination with the ulnar nerve palsy, would lead you to think about a lesion in the shoulder region affecting the brachial plexus. The combination of Horner's syndrome should raise the suspicion of a lesion interfering with preganglionic sympathetic fibres in the cervical sympathetic chain. If all this is put together, it is highly suspicious of a Pancoast tumour (Professor Henry Pancoast, American physician, 1932), a malignant tumour in the apex of the ipsilateral lung. Horner's syndrome, in the presence of shoulder pain, should always lead you to think of an apical lung cancer. Pancoast tumours are rare—less than 5% of lung cancers—and can be hard to spot as they often do not show up on X-ray. Therefore, a CT scan of the thorax, or sometimes an MRI scan, should be arranged if suspicion is high. Horner's syndrome can occur with dissection of the carotid artery, but in this case pain is usually facial and with an acute onset, so an MRI scan of the neck would be less helpful. Central lesions can also lead to it but are usually longer-standing and not associated with shoulder pain. Given that the bony pain is so localized, a bone scan would not be indicated. Nerve conduction studies may outline an ulnar nerve dysfunction but would not help find a cause.

→ http://www.cancerresearchuk.org/about-cancer/cancers-in-general/cancer-questions/what-is-a-pancoast-tumour

6. **B** ★★★

Allen's test assesses the integrity of the palmar arch and helps to identify patients in whom there would be additional risk of distal ischaemia associated with the insertion of a radial artery cannula, performance of radial arterial blood sampling, or harvest of radial artery for surgical grafting.

→ http://www.euro.who.int/__data/assets/pdf_file/0005/268790/WHO-guidelines-on-drawing-blood-best-practices-in-phlebotomy-Eng.pdf?ua=1

7. **D** ★★★   OHCS 10th edn → p. 755

Brown-Séquard syndrome describes a rare incomplete spinal cord lesion. It can present both in primary and secondary care as either an acute injury or as a consequence of disease such as a tumour or an infection. The clinical presentation is often a cause for difficulty due to hemisection of the cord and, as such, its effect on different tracts of the cord. Two key facts regarding the neurology need to be recalled in order to understand the clinical presentation: firstly, the crossover of the descending corticospinal tract (containing motor signals) and ascending dorsal columns (containing proprioception and fine touch input) occurs at the level of the medulla; also the ascending spinothalamic tracts (containing pain and temperature input) which cross one to two levels above their dorsal root at the spinal cord itself. An injury causing a hemisection of the cord will lead to loss of motor function, proprioception, and fine touch on the same side as those fibres have already crossed at a higher level. However, the contralateral pain and temperature sensation is affected for areas below the level, as they cross at the spinal cord itself. Any patient presenting with an incomplete spinal cord injury can be called a Brown-Séquard. However, not all patients present in the same way, depending on the exact cause and site of lesion. The syndrome was first described by Charles-Edouard Brown-Séquard who documented injuries in sugar cane farmers in Mauritius in the nineteenth century.

→ http://patient.info/doctor/brown-sequards-syndrome

8. C ★★★★

Ludwig's angina is a rare bacterial infection of the floor of the mouth, often associated with a dental abscess or recent oral trauma. It can progress rapidly and threaten airway patency, so it needs to be assessed and treated promptly.

→ https://medlineplus.gov/ency/article/001047.htm

9. B ★★★★ OHCS 10th edn → p. 644

This baby has typical features of a mucopolysaccharidosis (MPS) such as Hurler's (Gertrude Hurler, 1919) or Hunter's (Charles Hunter, 1917) syndrome. These cause a build-up of large sugar molecules—mucopolysaccharides, now known as glycosaminoglycans (GAGs)—in tissues in the body due to an enzyme deficiency. MPS 1—Hurler's—is autosomal recessive and MPS 2—Hunter's—is X-linked. Symptoms are progressive and range in severity. Severe forms present in the first year of life with features due to tissue build-up, e.g. organomegaly, skeletal deformity, coarse facial features and macroglossia, hernias, cardiomyopathy. In this child, the chest symptoms and poor feeding are likely due to the large tongue, bulbar dysfunction, and aspiration. Urine testing is a useful part of a metabolic work-up in children when an inborn error of metabolism is suspected. In this case, excess GAGs will leak out in the urine and give a clue to the diagnosis. White cell enzymes can then be tested for the specific enzyme defect. Urine amino acids will be generally elevated in renal disease. Organic acid patterns will be abnormal in organic acidaemias, such as methylmalonic acidaemia, where specific amino acids build up and leak out. Urine-reducing substances are non-glucose sugars that may leak out in the urine in disorders of sugar metabolism such as galactosaemia. Microscopic haematuria is found in a number of conditions, mostly involving the renal tract.

10. D ★★★★

Poland syndrome is a rare congenital defect characterized by under-developed or absence of the pectoralis muscles and ipsilateral syndactyly. Pectus excavatum is characterized by a depressed sternum, giving a concave appearance to the chest wall. Pectus carinatum, also known as pigeon chest, is a congenital defect with prominent sternum and ribs. Down's syndrome (trisomy 21) is a genetic disorder which is characterized by numerous physical and intellectual defects, one of which includes syndactyly.

11. A ★★★★   OHCS 10th edn → p. 166

Severe aortic regurgitation causes a number of eponymous signs, rarely seen nowadays.

→   https://en.wikipedia.org/wiki/Aortic_insufficiency#Signs_and_symptoms

12. D ★★★★

Gradenigo's syndrome describes the extension of a middle ear infection to the petrous apex. When this occurs, the patient is toxic and can develop an abducens nerve palsy from petrous apicitis and also pain behind the eye due to irritation of the ophthalmic branch of the trigeminal nerve. Ganser syndrome occurs when a person deliberately pretends to have a mental illness. Gilbert's syndrome is a genetic disorder with high levels of bilirubin leading to jaundice. Goldenhar syndrome, also known as OAV syndrome (oculo-auriculo-vertebral syndrome), is associated with abnormal facial development. Guillain–Barré syndrome is a progressive, immune-mediated, ascending peripheral neuropathy.

13. D ★★★★   OHCS 10th edn → p. 644

A Galeazzi fracture is a fracture of the distal radius with a dislocation of the distal radio-ulnar joint. Fractures of the ulna with radial head dislocations are described as a Monteggia fracture. A dorsally angulated fracture of the distal radius is commonly described as a Colles' fracture, and intra-articular fractures of the distal radius as a Barton's fracture.

Chapter 11

Orthopaedics

Nev Davies and Anuhya Vusirikala

Over the years, orthopaedic surgery has evolved into a vast specialty that is ever growing, with new technology, techniques, and implants. Computer-assisted surgery and minimally invasive approaches are current hot topics that are pushing the boundaries of what constitutes gold standard care for patients.

This specialty touches people of all ages from all walks of life. The practicality and logic in decision-making and management appeal to today's modern 'orthopods'.

Common paediatric orthopaedic conditions, such as developmental dysplasia of the hip and septic arthritis, can have serious consequences for the rest of the child's life if unrecognized and so are represented in this chapter.

Arthroplasty has been one of the true successes of the twenty-first century, and now over 160 000 knee and hip replacements are performed each year in the UK, revolutionizing the quality of life of patients with painful disabling arthritis.

To be a good orthopaedic surgeon requires not only a wide knowledge base, but also common sense, logic, and practical skills. 'A good surgeon knows how to operate; a great surgeon knows when to operate' is a classic saying that was drilled into me as a young houseman. In this specialty, there are often several management options facing the surgeon and the patient, and through careful discussion and the process of informed consent, a joint plan can be formulated and executed.

The questions in this chapter will help you to prepare both for your exams and for a future career as a doctor.

QUESTIONS

1. A 6-week-old baby with a 'clicky' hip is referred by the health visitor. She has had an ultrasound scan that confirms a dislocated right hip and a dysplastic acetabulum. Which single clinical finding best supports the diagnosis of a dislocated right hip? ★

A Asymmetrical skin creases on the thighs

B Clicking on abduction of the hip

C A dimple at the base of the spine

D Leg length discrepancy

E Limited abduction of the hip on the right

2. An 83-year-old man has had intermittent pain in the base of his spine for 4 months. It has become constant in nature and is not responding to simple analgesics. Which single factor in the history should alert you to the possibility of a serious pathology? ★

A Night pain

B Past history of malignancy

C Sciatic pain radiating down the leg from the buttock to the foot

D Scoliosis

E Temperature of 38°C or more

3. A 30-year-old woman who is usually fit and well has had intermittent urinary incontinence and loss of sensation around her bottom for the last 24 hours. Which is the single most appropriate next step in management? ★

A Blood tests, spinal X-rays, and a urine dipstick

B History and examination, including a rectal examination

C Mobilization of the theatre team, as she needs to go straight to theatre

D Opiate analgesia and review by senior colleagues

E Urgent magnetic resonance imaging (MRI) scan of the spine

4. A 7-year-old boy has had intermittent pain in his left hip for the past month. He walks with a slight limp and has decreased abduction at the hip joint. Which is the single most likely diagnosis? ★

A Juvenile idiopathic arthritis

B Missed developmental dysplasia of the hip

C Perthes' disease

D Slipped upper femoral epiphysis

E Transient synovitis

5. A 4-year-old boy has had pain and tenderness in his lower leg for 1 week. He is refusing to weight-bear. There is an area of swelling and warmth at the upper tibia which is tender. He has a temperature of 39°C. His blood tests show:

- white cell count 30 × 10⁹/L
- erythrocyte sedimentation rate (ESR) 110 mm/hour
- C-reactive protein (CRP) 200 mg/L.

Which is the single most likely causative microorganism? ★

A *Kingella kingae*

B *Pseudomonas aeruginosa*

C *Salmonella paratyphi*

D *Staphylococcus aureus*

E *Staphylococcus epidermidis*

6. A 70-year-old woman with rheumatoid arthritis is having a total knee replacement. Which is the single most important preoperative investigation? ★

A Anteroposterior and lateral radiographs of the cervical spine

B Arterial blood gas analysis

C Dual-energy X-ray absorptiometry (DEXA) scanning

D Inflammatory markers

E Up-to-date anteroposterior and lateral X-rays of the knee

7. A newborn baby has 'clicky' hips at birth. Which single feature is a risk factor for developmental dysplasia of the hip (DDH)? ★

A Family history of DDH

B Low birthweight

C Male gender

D Polyhydramnios

E Second sibling

8. A 45-year-old builder has pins and needles down the medial border of his forearm and weakness in the small muscles in his hand, causing him to drop things. Which is the single name and location of the nerve that is being compressed? ★

A Anterior interosseous nerve under the fibres of the flexor digitorum sublimis

B Median nerve in the carpal tunnel

C Posterior interosseous nerve under the proximal edge of the supinator muscle

D Ulnar nerve at the cubital tunnel

E Ulnar nerve in Guyon's canal

9. A 65-year-old man sustained a fracture of the femoral neck 4 years ago. He is undergoing a total hip replacement for collapse of the head and secondary osteoarthritis. He walks with a stick and has an antalgic gait and a significant leg length discrepancy. Which is the single most likely benefit of the procedure? ★

A Equalization of the leg length discrepancy

B Improvement of walking distance

C Improvement of range of motion

D Pain relief

E Prevention of compensatory osteoarthritis in other joints

10. A 60-year-old man has a deformed painless right ankle and foot. He has had blistering and ulceration of his foot in the past. X-rays show a destructive Charcot-type arthropathy of the ankle and subtalar joints. Which is the single most likely underlying diagnosis? ★

A Alcohol-induced peripheral neuropathy

B Diabetes mellitus

C Hereditary motor and sensory neuropathy

D Leprosy

E Tertiary syphilis

11. A 75-year-old man attends his 6-week follow-up appointment after a primary right total hip replacement for osteoarthritis. He walks in with the aid of one stick and, as he walks, his upper body sways to the right when he stands on his operated leg. Which is the single best description of his altered gait? ★

A Antalgic

B Normal for this stage in his post-operative recovery

C Short leg

D Trendelenburg positive

E Varus thrust

12. A 36-year-old computer programmer has a painful lump on the volar aspect of his wrist. The lump is well defined, fluctuant, and pulsatile, but it does not transilluminate. Which is the single most appropriate next step in management? ★

A Aspirate the lump in the clinic under local anaesthesia, and inject steroid

B Explain the benign nature of the lump and that it is likely to resolve spontaneously with time

C Organize an ultrasound scan to confirm the diagnosis

D Put the patient on the waiting list for excision of the lump under general anaesthesia

E Put the patient on the waiting list for excision of the lump under local anaesthesia

13. A 60-year-old woman has sustained a low-energy fracture of the distal radius. Last year, she fell and sustained a proximal femoral fracture, which was fixed with a dynamic hip screw. A recent dual-energy X-ray absorptiometry (DEXA) scan has shown a T score of –3. Which is the single most likely diagnosis? ★ ★

A Oligodystrophy

B Osteomalacia

C Osteopenia

D Osteopetrosis

E Osteoporosis

14. A patient is concerned about the risk of deep infection following a primary total hip replacement. Which single factor has had the greatest impact on reducing joint replacement infection? ★ ★

A Antibiotic-loaded cement

B Body-exhaust suits for the surgeons

C Disposable gowns

D Laminar air flow systems

E Peri-operative prophylactic systemic antibiotics

15. A 60-year-old woman has had neck pain for several years. She now has an acute prolapse of the C5/6 disc, causing nerve root compression on the right side. Which single set of symptoms and signs is she most likely to have? ★ ★

A Dysaesthesia in the thumb and index finger, and weakness of elbow extension

B Increased tone and hyper-reflexia in the right arm

C None of these

D Pain and numbness in the medial forearm

E Weakness of elbow flexion and loss of triceps reflex

16. A 2-year-old girl has had multiple bony fractures since birth. She has discoloured teeth, poor growth, and blue sclera. Which is the single most likely diagnosis? ★ ★

A Achondroplasia

B Craniocleidodysostosis

C Hypophosphatasia

D Osteogenesis imperfecta

E Osteopetrosis

17. A 50-year-old man has increasing pain in his right knee. The pain is not controlled by daily ibuprofen and paracetamol, and he is particularly troubled by it when going up and down stairs. He experiences pain even when at rest. He had a total meniscectomy 30 years ago after a football injury when he also ruptured his anterior cruciate ligament. His X-ray is shown in Figure 11.1 (see Colour Plate section). Which is the single most appropriate management? ★ ★

A Increase his pain medications and advise him to use a stick

B Medial unicompartmental knee replacement

C Referral for physiotherapy

D Steroid injection and review

E Total knee replacement

18. A baby has been born with a foot deformity, as shown in Figure 11.2 (see Colour Plate section). Which is the single best description of this foot deformity? ★ ★

A Calcaneus, abductus, valgus

B Cavus, adductus, varus, equinus

C Cavus, calcaneus, adductus, varus

D Cavus, valgus, equinus

E Pes planus

19. A 26-year-old man who plays squash socially presents with a 4-month history of unilateral heel pain. He has circumferential thickening of the Achilles tendon, 2 cm proximal to its insertion at the os calcis, and is unable to perform a tiptoe test. Which is the single most likely diagnosis? ★ ★

A Achilles insertional tendonitis

B Chronic Achilles tendon rupture

C Hagland's deformity of the os calcis

D Retrocalcaneal bursitis

E Tibialis posterior tendonitis

20. A 15-year old boy presents to the orthopaedic paediatric clinic with a 3-month history of pain and swelling in his right thigh. He has also reported night sweats and recent weight loss. An X-ray of his right thigh shows a large lesion in the diaphysis of his femur with an onion skin appearance. A needle biopsy is performed, and the histological evaluation shows small, round blue cells. Which is the single most likely diagnosis? ★ ★ ★ ★

A Chrondrosarcoma

B Ewing's sarcoma

C Osteochondroma

D Osteosarcoma

E Osteoid osteoma

21. A 60-year-old man has an acutely painful, swollen knee. In total, 100 mL of synovial fluid is aspirated. The fluid is straw-coloured and viscous. Analysis shows no crystals and a white cell count of 4000/mm^3 with neutrophils <25%. The patient reports that his pain is much improved after aspiration. Which is the single most likely diagnosis? ★ ★ ★ ★

A Gout

B Pseudogout

C Reactive arthritis

D Rheumatoid arthritis

E Septic arthritis

22. A 65-year-old man has undergone a primary total hip replacement for osteoarthritis. Post-operatively, he has developed a foot drop, with numbness in his foot and weakness of ankle dorsiflexion to 2/5 power. Which is the single most likely cause of the foot drop? ★ ★ ★ ★

A Axonotmesis of the common peroneal nerve at the head of the fibula due to pressure from positioning during the procedure

B Axonotmesis of the sciatic nerve due to intra-operative traction injury secondary to misplaced retractors

C Neuropraxia of the common peroneal nerve at the head of the fibula due to pressure from positioning during the procedure

D Neuropraxia of the sciatic nerve due to intra-operative traction injury secondary to misplaced retractors

E Neurotmesis of the sciatic nerve during surgery

23. A 13-year-old boy has had repeated ankle sprains, mid-foot pain, and problems walking on uneven ground. He has a flat foot that does not correct into varus when he stands on tiptoe. He also has a stiff subtalar joint. Which is the single most likely diagnosis? ★ ★ ★ ★

A Charcot–Marie–Tooth disease

B Lateral ligament insufficiency (ankle)

C Physiological flexible flat foot

D Sever's disease

E Tarsal coalition

24. A 50-year-old diabetic man has recurrent triggering of the ring finger. The finger is stuck in flexion. It was injected 2 years ago, with good results. Which is the single most appropriate management? ★ ★ ★ ★

A Operative release under general anaesthesia

B Operative release under local anaesthesia

C Repeat of the injection

D Stretching and a night splint with physiotherapy

E Ultrasound scan to confirm the diagnosis

ANSWERS

1. E ★   OHCS 10th edn → pp. 686–7

Clicking and asymmetry of skin creases are 'soft' signs of hip dislocation. The limitation of abduction of the hip suggests a positive Ortolani's test, which means that the hip is out of joint posteriorly.

2. B ★   OHCS 10th edn → p. 680

This suggests that spinal metastases may be the cause. The other features may also be present with metastatic lesions but can be features of other diagnoses. Night pain can indicate significant pathology and should be taken seriously.

3. B ★   OHCS 10th edn → p. 681

This history suggests cauda equina syndrome, of which there are many causes. However, the young age makes a sinister cause unlikely. The first step is always a thorough history and examination, and a rectal examination must always be performed to assess anal tone.

4. C ★   OHCS 10th edn → p. 684

In this age group, the most important cause of persistent limp is Perthes' disease, which is an avascular necrosis of the femoral head. Slipped upper femoral epiphysis tends to occur in older overweight children. Transient synovitis should not last for a month. Dysplasia of the hip would have been seen at an earlier age than 7 years. All children in the UK have their hips checked at birth, at 6 weeks, at 8 months, and at 2 years. Juvenile idiopathic arthritis is possible but less likely.

5. D ★   OHCS 10th edn → p. 696

This is a picture of osteomyelitis, commonly caused by *Staphylococcus aureus*.

6. A ★   OHCS 10th edn → pp. 614–15

Guidelines exist that recommend which preoperative investigations should be performed. However, patients with rheumatoid arthritis are at risk of cervical involvement, which can make anaesthetic management of the neck and airway difficult. If in doubt, always discuss the case with an anaesthetist.

→ https://www.nice.org.uk/guidance/NG45 (routine preoperative tests for elective surgery)

7. A ★   OHCS 10th edn → pp. 686–7

The risk factors for DDH are as follows:

- female gender
- first born

- foot first (breech)
- family history
- further bony abnormalities (e.g. talipes equinovarus).

8. D ★   OHCS 10th edn → p. 669

The ulnar nerve is responsible for the sensory and motor presentation of this problem. The ulnar nerve passes through the cubital tunnel at the elbow, whereas Guyon's canal is at the wrist. Compression at Guyon's canal could not account for the symptoms.

9. D ★   OHCS 10th edn → p. 704

The main benefit of hip replacement is pain control. It is much less successful in improving mobility.

10. B ★

This patient's age makes hereditary motor and sensory neuropathy unlikely. Diabetes is the commonest cause of neuropathy, leading to arthropathy.

11. D ★   OHCS 10th edn → p. 682

The Trendelenburg test assesses the stability of the hip. When the patient stands on the affected leg, the pelvis falls on the opposite side, causing the upper body to lurch to the affected side in order to compensate. This is a positive test. It is caused by weak abductor muscles, a dislocated hip, or the absence of a stable fulcrum.

12. C ★   OHCS 10th edn → p. 670

This is the classic location and description of a ganglion, i.e. a benign bulge of the synovium. It may resolve spontaneously, but if it is painful, it can be aspirated or excised. However, diagnosis should be confirmed first with soft tissue imaging.

13. E ★★

DEXA stands for dual-energy X-ray absorptiometry and is considered to be the most accurate test for bone density. Although standard X-rays show changes in bone density after about 40% bone loss, a DEXA scan can detect changes after about a 1% change. The results of a DEXA scan are reported in two ways—as T scores and as Z scores. A T score compares the bone density with the optimal peak bone density for gender. It is reported as the number of standard deviations below the mean. A T score of greater than −1 is considered to be normal. A T score of −1 to −2.5 is considered to be osteopenia and the patient is at risk of developing osteoporosis. A T score of less than −2.5 is diagnostic of osteoporosis. A Z score compares the patient's bone density with that of someone of the same age.

14. E ★★

To prevent surgical site infections, antibiotic prophylaxis should be given before:

- clean surgery involving the placement of a prosthesis or implant
- clean-contaminated surgery
- contaminated surgery. → https://www.nice.org.uk/guidance/cg74 (surgical site infections: prevention and treatment)

15. A ★★   OHCS 10th edn → pp. 660, 716–17

Knowledge of the specific patterns of nerve damage is useful in diagnosis (see the tables and pictures in OHCS 10th edn).

16. D ★★

These are the features of some types of osteogenesis imperfecta, a rare cause of multiple fractures. These signs may help to raise suspicion of the diagnosis.

17. E ★★   OHCS 10th edn → p. 704

For this patient, non-operative measures for the management of his osteoarthritis have been exhausted, and surgical treatment is warranted. His X-ray shows medial compartment osteoarthritis. However, he requires a total knee replacement because a unicompartmental knee replacement is contraindicated in a patient without an anterior cruciate ligament.

18. B ★★   OHCS 10th edn → p. 686

This is an image of club foot, or talipes equinovarus. A full club foot involves the ankle (talus) and foot (pes), and is equinus (the heel is elevated like that of a horse) and cavus (with an exaggerated arch). It is varus (turned inward) and adducted (moved towards the midline). It cannot be moved through the normal range of movements, and the Achilles tendon is tight and the calf muscle shortened.

19. B ★★

This question requires you to correctly identify the Achilles tendon as the source of the pathology. Patients with tibialis posterior tendonitis also find it difficult to stand on tiptoe. Circumferential thickening could be due to chronic rupture or tendonitis. Retrocalcaneal bursitis tenderness tends to be located more distally, behind the tendon.

20. B ★★★★   OHCS 10th edn → p. 698

Ewing's sarcoma is the second commonest primary malignant bone tumour in children. These tumours are found in the diaphysis of long bones. Based on the history, radiological appearance (periosteal reaction may give an onion skin or sunburst appearance), and histology, the patient has Ewing's sarcoma.

21. C ★★★★ OHCS 10th edn → pp. 706–7

Analysis of the colour, viscosity, and composition of the synovial fluid is important. In this patient, the straw colour and high viscosity, but low number of neutrophils point to a non-inflammatory cause. In patients with inflammation or infection, the fluid is yellow with a high number of neutrophils.

22. D ★★★★ OHCS 10th edn → p. 705

Neuropraxia (physiological conduction block) is the commonest type of nerve injury encountered, usually due to compression on the nerve. In total hip replacement, misplaced retractors are the usual cause of this, and the sciatic nerve is the most commonly involved nerve. Neuropraxia is often explained to patients as 'bruising to the nerve'. Nerve function usually returns to normal, although this can take many months.

23. E ★★★★

Tarsal coalition—an abnormal connection between the tarsal bones—commonly presents in adolescence as the connection ossifies with growth of the child. Often there is a history of repeated ankle sprains and difficulty walking on uneven ground.

24. B ★★★★ OHCS 10th edn → p. 670

Diabetics are renowned for having recurrent resistant triggering digits. Operative release under local anaesthesia avoids the complications of general anaesthesia (which are increased in a diabetic patient) and allows the surgeon to check the release by asking the patient to move the finger intra-operatively.

Chapter 12

Trauma

Nev Davies and Anuhya Vusirikala

Trauma is a major public health problem and it is the commonest cause of death in those under the age of 40. Trauma care is a multidisciplinary specialty, and orthopaedic surgeons play an essential role in the initial and definitive management of patients with musculoskeletal injuries—saving lives and saving limb.

The care provided to seriously injured trauma patients has improved significantly for a variety of reasons, including enhanced pre-hospital input, provision of care within a network of Major Trauma Units, and the availability of specialist rehabilitation services in hospital and in the community. The primary aim of the trauma team is to rapidly assess, resuscitate, and stabilize trauma patients and determine the extent of injuries sustained, so that the most appropriate immediate treatment can be administered.

The questions in this chapter will highlight the important principles of trauma care and help you better comprehend the management of a seriously injured trauma patient.

QUESTIONS

1. A 17-year-old man is knocked off his moped. He is wearing a helmet, and witnesses thought that he was travelling at 30 mph before impact. Which is the single most appropriate immediate management? ★

A Advanced Trauma Life Support (ATLS) assessment following guidelines

B Computed tomography (CT) scan of his head

C Glasgow Coma Scale assessment and pupil reaction

D Thorough mechanism of injury history and full examination

E X-rays of his chest, pelvis, and cervical spine

2. A motorcyclist has been involved in a motor vehicle collision. He is talking and has bruising on the right side of his chest but normal breath sounds; his pulse rate is 120 bpm, and his blood pressure is 60/40 mmHg. His Glasgow Coma Scale score is 15/15. He has bruising around his flanks and an obvious open fracture of his right tibia. He has blood at the urethral meatus. His chest X-ray shows some fractured ribs on the right, and his pelvic film is shown in Figure 12.1 (see Colour Plate section). Which is the single most appropriate next step in his management? ★

A Betadine-soaked dressing, intravenous (IV) antibiotics, and washout of his tibial fracture

B Chest drain for his rib fractures and potential haemothorax

C IV access, IV fluids, and blood replacement

D Pelvic external fixation

E Securing of a definitive airway with the anaesthetist

3. A 6-year-old boy is brought to the Emergency Department with a painful swollen arm. His mother is unsure what happened and gives a story of an unwitnessed fall off a bunk bed the day before. The boy has a lot of bruising all over his arm and upper body. Which is the single most appropriate management? ★

A Admit the child to the ward and contact your consultant

B Contact the duty social worker

C Discuss your concerns with the paediatrician on call

D Probe the mother about the cause of the bruises

E Send off a full blood count and clotting screen

4. A 9-year-old boy has put his arm through a glass door. There is significant bleeding from a 5-cm deep wound in his forearm. Which is the single most appropriate immediate management? ★

A Apply a high arm tourniquet

B Apply direct pressure over the axillary artery

C Apply direct pressure over the wound

D Give intravenous (IV) antibiotics and tetanus prophylaxis

E Give local anaesthetic and clip the bleeding vessel

5. A 25-year-old man has been involved in a drunken brawl and has been stabbed in the chest. His respiratory rate is 25 breaths/minute, heart rate 110 bpm, and blood pressure 85/60 mmHg. He has two wounds in the left thorax. Which is the single most appropriate immediate management? ★

A Apply direct pressure over the stab wounds to stem the bleeding

B Fast bleep the cardiothoracic surgeons

C Obtain intravenous (IV) access and cross-match 6 units of blood

D Open the airway and give high-flow oxygen

E Open the chest (thoracotomy) and begin internal cardiac massage

6. A 7-year-old boy has an open fracture of his forearm. He is on a scout trip away from home and attends the hospital with his scout leader. You need to take him to theatre immediately but are unable to contact his parents who are away on holiday. Which is the single most appropriate course of action? ★

A Ask a duty social worker to sign the consent form

B Ask another doctor to sign the consent form

C Ask the boy to sign the consent form

D Ask the scout leader to sign the consent form

E Written consent is not required as this is an emergency

7. A 25-year-old man has been knocked off his motorcycle. He has an open fracture of his femur. His leg X-ray is shown in Figure 12.2 (see Colour Plate section). Which is the single most appropriate definitive management? ★ ★

A External fixator with washout and debridement of the wound and delayed primary closure

B Intramedullary nail with washout and debridement of the wound and delayed primary closure

C Open reduction and plate fixation with washout and debridement of the wound and primary closure

D Washout and debridement of the wound and application of a Thomas splint

E Washout and debridement of the wound and a long leg cast with a window for a vacuum suction pump

8. A 79-year-old woman has fallen at home. She has hip pain and a short, externally rotated left leg. Radiographs show a displaced intracapsular fracture of her left neck of femur. Previously she walked outdoors independently with the aid of a stick. She is otherwise medically fit. Which is the single most appropriate surgical management? ★ ★

A Cemented hemiarthroplasty

B Dynamic hip screw and plate

C Total hip replacement

D Uncemented hemiarthroplasty

E Three divergent cannulated screws

9. A 35-year-old man, who was injured in a road traffic accident, is admitted to the Emergency Department. His eyes open to painful stimuli and he moans periodically. His left arm is deformed and does not respond to painful stimuli, but his right arm purposefully moves towards the painful stimulus. Which is the single most appropriate Glasgow Coma Scale (GCS) score for this patient? ★ ★ ★

A 4

B 5

C 8

D 9

E 13

10. A 75-year-old man sustained a head injury following a fall, sustaining a 3-cm scalp laceration. In the Emergency Department, he appears mildly confused, with a Glasgow Coma Scale (GCS) score of 14. His heart rate is 85 bpm and his blood pressure is 135/70 mmHg. He has had one episode of vomiting in hospital. He is currently on warfarin for atrial fibrillation but is otherwise well. Which is the single most appropriate initial management? ★ ★ ★

A Admit for head injury observations

B Check ethanol levels

C Perform a computed tomography (CT) scan of his head

D Skull X-ray

E Suture the scalp laceration

11. A 20-year-old man falls off his motorbike and fractures his tibial shaft. The management options are discussed with him and he opts for an intramedullary nail. He is put into a backslab cast and listed for surgery the next day. His leg is kept strictly elevated. At 3.30 a.m., he develops increasing pain despite morphine treatment. Which is the single most appropriate next step in management? ★ ★ ★

A Add a non-steroidal anti-inflammatory drug to his pain relief, and review in 30 minutes

B Call the anaesthetist to set up a patient-controlled morphine analgesia system

C Call your senior colleague, as the patient needs to go to theatre immediately

D List the patient for theatre at 6 a.m., when his stomach will be empty and it will be safe to give him an anaesthetic

E Split his cast to skin, continue elevation, and review him with a senior colleague in 15 minutes

12. A 93-year-old woman is bed-bound in a nursing home and has severe dementia. She has fallen out of bed. Her right hip is stiff but painless, and an X-ray reveals a dislocated total hip replacement (THR). She also has a large 10 × 5 cm open pre-tibial laceration. She has a respiratory rate of 23 breaths/minute, with evidence of ischaemic changes on the electrocardiogram (ECG). Which is the single most appropriate specialty to call for help with the management of this patient? ★ ★ ★

A Anaesthetist, to give a general anaesthetic to reduce the THR

B Cardiologist, to help to interpret the ECG changes

C General medical team, to optimize medical care prior to any intervention

D Plastic surgeon, to help to manage the open pre-tibial laceration

E Psychiatrist, to assess whether the patient can consent to treatment

13. A 6-year-old boy has a fall onto his left outstretched hand. He now has difficulty in pronating his forearm, flexing his wrist and thumb. He also complains about loss of sensation in the lateral palm and radial three-and-a-half digits. His X-ray shows a supracondylar fracture of the left humerus. Which is the single most likely nerve that is damaged? ★★★

A Anterior interosseous branch of the median nerve

B Deep branch of the radial nerve

C Palmar cutaneous branch of the median nerve

D Superficial branch of the radial nerve

E Ulnar nerve

14. A 35-year-old man was playing five-a-side football when he thought he had been kicked in the back of the leg. The next day he is hobbling and has pain and swelling around his Achilles tendon. Simmonds' test is equivocal. Which is the single most appropriate investigation to confirm the diagnosis and plan further management? ★★★★

A Computed tomography (CT) scan

B Examination under anaesthesia

C Magnetic resonance imaging (MRI) scan

D Plain X-ray

E Ultrasound scan

15. A 25-year-old man with epilepsy has a painful swollen shoulder after having a fit earlier that day. X-rays are taken and shown in Figure 12.3 (see Colour Plate section). Which is the single most appropriate management? ★★★★

A Arrange for a computed tomography (CT) scan to help to plan operative management

B Arrange for the patient to go to theatre for a closed reduction

C Arrange for the patient to go to theatre for an open reduction

D Perform reduction using the Hippocratic method under sedation

E Perform reduction using Kocher's method under sedation

16. A 45-year-old woman has an oblique fracture of her distal fibula. Which is the single best technique to compress the two fragments of bone? ★★★★

A Dynamic compression plate and cancellous screws

B Elastic titanium intramedullary nails

C External fixation with supplementary K-wire fixation

D Lag screw and neutralization plate

E Locking plate with locking screws

17. A 45-year-old man has fallen 20 feet off a ladder. As he fell, his right leg became caught in the rungs of the ladder and he felt his knee 'pop in and pop out'. He has a very swollen, tender knee, with a cool, white limb and a very faint dorsalis pedis pulse. Which is the single most appropriate immediate management? ★ ★ ★ ★

A Anteroposterior and lateral lower limb radiographs

B Mobilize the theatre team immediately, as the patient needs to undergo an open exploration of the popliteal vessels

C Magnetic resonance imaging (MRI) of the patient's knee to determine which ligaments are damaged

D Organize an arteriogram and contact the vascular surgeons for an urgent review

E Organize an urgent fasciotomy to prevent compartment syndrome

18. A 15-year-old boy has fractured his humerus. His X-ray is shown in Figure 12.4 (see Colour Plate section). Which is the single most likely mechanism of injury? ★ ★ ★ ★

A Bending force

B Bending force with axial compression

C Direct impact from the lateral aspect

D Direct impact from the medial aspect

E Torsional force

19. A 22-year-old footballer ruptures his anterior cruciate ligament and tears his medial meniscus after twisting his knee in training. Which single group of clinical findings is most likely 2 weeks after the initial injury? ★ ★ ★ ★

A Effusion, hyperextension, and generalized joint line tenderness

B Effusion, medial joint line tenderness, and positive Lachman's test

C Increased opening on valgus stress, and tenderness medially

D Increased posterior sag, positive anterior draw, and negative Lachman's test

E Quadriceps wasting, extensor lag, and positive Lachman's test

ANSWERS

1. A ★   OHCS 10th edn → p. 781

The ATLS guidelines are regarded as the international gold standard for the initial management of the traumatized patient.

→ https://www.rcseng.ac.uk/education-and-exams/courses/search/advanced-trauma-life-support-atls-provider-programme/

2. C ★

In keeping with any significant injury, as per the Advanced Trauma Life Support (ATLS) principles, the immediate priority is to ensure that airway, breathing, and circulation are not compromised. This man's airway and breathing seem to be secure, as determined by a normal Glasgow Coma Scale score and the ability to phonate, so you should go on to treat the potential blood loss from the pelvic fracture by securing circulation.

3. C ★   OHCS 10th edn → p. 146

Any doctor who sees children needs to be aware of the possibility of non-accidental injury. However, although it is important to document exactly what you have found, specialist paediatric doctors should be involved in these cases. They can work with the parent specialty team to gather further information and plan appropriate management.

4. C ★

Following the ABC (airway, breathing, and circulation) guidelines, the first step in controlling bleeding is the application of direct pressure. Once the bleeding is under control, this patient may need further surgical intervention, and antibiotics and tetanus prophylaxis may be indicated, but these are not the priorities.

5. D ★

Following the Advanced Trauma Life Support (ATLS) guidelines, securing an airway is always the first priority.

6. E ★

Only a person with parental responsibility can give valid consent on behalf of a child who is not Gillick-competent. In some cases, the parent may sign over parental responsibility to another adult, but usually this does not happen. In an emergency, the doctor should document the need for an emergency procedure clearly and state why it is needed, but can proceed to save life or limb without formal written consent.

→ http://www.gmc-uk.org/guidance/ethical_guidance/children_guidance_index.asp (*Good medical practice: 0–18 years: guidance for all doctors*)

7. B ★★   OHCS 10th edn → pp. 734–5

Intramedullary nails align and stabilize the bone and share the load with the bone. They allow early mobilization. Because the fracture is open, it requires careful washing out. Delayed primary closure refers to the initial debridement and then closing of the wound at a later stage. This allows better healing of contaminated wounds.

→ https://www.boa.ac.uk/wp-content/uploads/2014/12/BOAST-4.pdf (BOAST 4 guideline: the management of severe open lower limb fractures)

8. C ★★

Intracapsular fractures require either a total hip replacement or a hemiarthroplasty. Patients who were able to walk independently outside with the aid of no more than a stick, who are not cognitively impaired, and who are medically fit for anaesthesia and surgery should be offered a total hip replacement.

→ http://guidance.nice.org.uk/CG124 (National Institute for Health and Care Excellence (2011). Hip fracture: management. NICE clinical guideline, CG124)

9. D ★★★

It is important to be able to calculate the Glasgow Coma Scale score in critically ill patients. This patient has a score of 9:

- eye opening—2
- best verbal response—2
- best motor response—5. An abbreviated coma scale—AVPU—can be used for a quick initial assessment of a patient:[*]
- A—alert
- V—responds to voice
- P—responds to pain
- U—unresponsive.

→ http://www.glasgowcomascale.org/

10. C ★★★

As per the National Institute for Health and Care Excellence (NICE) guidelines on head injury, a computed tomography (CT) head would be the priority in this patient because of the following reasons:

- mildly confused with a GCS score of 14 since injury
- one episode of vomiting
- on warfarin therapy for atrial fibrillation.

* Source data from *Annals of Emergency Medicine*, 44, 2, Kelly CA, Upex A, Bateman DN, Comparison of consciousness level assessment in the poisoned patient using the alert/verbal/painful/unresponsive scale and the Glasgow Coma Scale, pp. 108–113.

11. E ★★★   OHCS 10th edn → p. 722

Patients with leg fractures are at risk of developing compartment syndrome, inflammation, and swelling within a closed fascial compartment, leading to an impaired blood supply. However, this man is in a cast, so simple relief of the external pressure and elevation may alleviate the pain and swelling. If the pain continues, he may be developing compartment syndrome and require fasciotomy, so a close review is essential.

12. C ★★★

This situation is not uncommon. The patient is more likely to suffer harm as a result of her medical illness than in relation to her dislocated THR, and medical problems should be co-managed with medical teams in the interest of best outcome for the patient.

Ortho-geriatricians are medically trained doctors who work closely with orthopaedic doctors to provide exactly this kind of input.

13. A ★★★   OHCS 10th edn → p. 727

The anterior interosseous branch (AIN) of the median nerve is the most commonly damaged nerve in supracondylar fractures. The AIN supplies the deep muscles of the forearm (flexor pollicis longus, lateral half of the flexor digitorum profundus, pronator quadratus). Damage to the AIN results in loss of pronation of the forearm, weakness in wrist flexion, and inability to flex the thumb. As his fracture is above the origin of the palmar cutaneous branch, there is loss of sensation in the lateral palm and the radial three-and-a-half digits.

14. E ★★★★   OHCS 10th edn → p. 712

A ruptured Achilles tendon causes sudden pain when running or jumping, and the heel cannot be raised from the floor when the patient is standing on the affected leg. In Simmonds' test, the patient kneels on a chair and the calf is squeezed; there will be less plantar flexion of the foot on the affected side. An ultrasound scan is the easiest and most discriminatory test for soft tissue injuries, although it is operator-dependent.

15. A ★★★★   OHCS 10th edn → p. 724

The radiographs show a locked posterior dislocation of the glenohumeral joint. This injury is often missed, as the signs (positive 'light-bulb' sign) are subtle in the anteroposterior view. The diagnosis is obvious in the axillary view. This is a difficult problem, and often further imaging is necessary to plan surgical management.

16. D ★★★★   OHCS 10th edn → p. 738

A lag screw is the best technique for producing interfragmentary compression in the context of absolute stability. This allows the fracture to heal by primary bone healing without the formation of a callus.

17. D ★★★★ OHCS 10th edn → p. 737

The history and examination findings should alert you to a possible knee dislocation that has self-reduced. This poses a significant risk to the neurovascular bundle. An arteriogram is the gold standard investigation, with an urgent review by the vascular surgeons.

18. E ★★★★

This is a spiral fracture, which is caused by a twisting force.

19. B ★★★★ OHCS 10th edn → pp. 688–9

This patient is likely to have a residual effusion 2 weeks after a significant knee injury. Joint line tenderness is a non-specific examination finding in a knee with intra-articular damage. Lachman's test, performed with the knee in 30° of flexion, is the most sensitive clinical test for diagnosing an anterior cruciate ligament injury. Important points are to compare with the other knee and the presence or absence of an end point.

Emergency medicine

Catherine Roberts

Emergency medicine is not all 'ER'—glamour and fast-moving action; much of it requires caring for relatively minor problems or complex elderly patients. Emergency Departments are busy, high-intensity work environments with a high turnover of patients. In order to make time-critical decisions effectively, it is necessary to have a good breadth and depth of knowledge underpinning a sensible and safe approach to dealing with clinical uncertainty. Patients will present with acute and chronic conditions from all specialties.

Gathering information rapidly is important. Gaining clues from the patient and their relative(s) is useful, as is obtaining information on events at the scene from the ambulance paramedics. Hospital notes are often not available and neither is the general practitioner (GP), so decisions are made on the basis of limited information. Rather than making definitive diagnoses confirmed by expensive tests, the role of the emergency physician is to determine the immediate threat to life or limb and to treat that threat, while gathering information to make a 'most likely' diagnosis so that treatment can be started. Observing the patient in a Clinical Decision Unit can often help to confirm your suspicions, give you further information on how severe a condition is, or eliminate a possible diagnosis.

Ultimately, emergency medicine requires the assessment of risk, evaluation of the added benefit of admission over discharge, and excellent communication. The only way to learn emergency medicine is to practise, to discuss patients, and to develop your analytical and decision-making skills. The following questions are designed to develop some of these skills, by showing you an approach to solving the clinical problems that are commonly encountered in the Emergency Department, how to use tests efficiently and effectively, and some of the options for treatment that are available other than admission under inpatient teams.

QUESTIONS

1. A 24-year-old man is hit by a car travelling at 50 mph. He is unconscious at the scene and there are only two rescuers. He has an obvious fracture of his right leg and swelling of his abdomen. Which is the single most appropriate immediate management of this patient's assumed cervical spine injury at the scene? ★

A Halo traction

B Manual in-line immobilization

C Manual in-line traction

D Semi-rigid cervical collar, blocks, and tape

E Soft sponge collar

2. A 46-year-old woman is in a coma. Her partner tells you that she has had abdominal pain and vomiting for 3 days. She is clinically dehydrated. Her blood sugar level is 48 mmol/L and her arterial pH is 7.0. An anaesthetist is present and managing her airway. Which is the single most appropriate immediate management? ★

A A 500 mL bolus of 0.9% saline

B Infusion of short-acting insulin at 10 U/hour

C Intravenous (IV) cyclizine

D IV piperacillin/tazobactam (Tazocin®)

E Normal saline 2 L with potassium 40 mmol/L over 4 hours

3. A 45-year-old man has a 2-cm laceration to the radial border of the middle and distal phalanges of his right index finger. Which is the single most appropriate local anaesthetic to use to close the wound? ★

A 0.5% bupivacaine without adrenaline (epinephrine)

B 1% lidocaine with adrenaline (epinephrine) 1:1000

C 1% lidocaine without adrenaline (epinephrine)

D 2% lidocaine with adrenaline (epinephrine) 1:1000

E 5% prilocaine without adrenaline (epinephrine)

4. A 40-year-old woman has pain and discharge from her right ear, a temperature of 38.3°C, a blocked nose, and a mild cough. She had slight pain and deafness in her right ear 1 week ago, which she treated with warm olive oil dripped into her ear. She is a tele-banking operator who uses a headset with an earpiece in her right ear. Which is the single most likely diagnosis? ★

A Extensive wax in the ear

B Foreign body in the ear

C Otitis externa

D Otitis media

E Perforated eardrum

5. A 56-year-old man has had a fall. He has a fracture of the radial head, which is undisplaced. Which is the single most appropriate method of immobilizing this fracture? ★

A Above-arm back slab

B Broad arm sling

C Collar and cuff

D Futura splint

E High arm sling

6. An 85-year-old man has an epistaxis. He is on warfarin for atrial fibrillation and his international normalized ratio (INR) is 6. Which single drug that he has recently been started on is most likely to be related to the cause of the epistaxis? ★

A Aspirin

B Bendroflumethiazide

C Clopidogrel

D Erythromycin

E Penicillin

7. An 89-year-old woman has had multiple falls. She has been to the Emergency Department 30 times in the last 6 months but has only been admitted once. You assess her and can find little acutely wrong with her, but are concerned about sending her home. She appears to be unsteady on her feet. Which single service would be most helpful in contributing to a management plan? ★

A General practitioner (GP)

B Hospital chiropody

C Hospital optician

D Medical registrar

E Occupational therapy

8. A 72-year-old man is brought to the Emergency Department in shock. His systolic blood pressure is 76 mmHg, with a pulse rate of 120 bpm. He has a history of 'coffee ground' vomiting and has melaena on rectal examination. Which is the single most appropriate immediate management? ★

A Application of a military anti-shock trouser (MAST) suit

B Intravenous (IV) bolus of gelofusine

C IV bolus of 5% dextrose

D IV infusion of noradrenaline (norepinephrine)

E Transfusion of packed red blood cells

9. A 27-year-old man has a sudden onset of severe occipital headache. Which single clinical sign is of greatest concern? ★

A Loss of consciousness

B Neck stiffness

C Photophobia

D Unilateral pain

E Vomiting

10. A 45-year-old man has a systolic blood pressure of 50 mmHg and a pulse rate of 120 bpm. Which single vascular access line would be the best to use? ★

A Green Venflon (18G)

B Grey Venflon (16G)

C Intraosseus needle

D Single-lumen central line

E Triple-lumen central line

11. A 45-year-old scaffolder has fallen 30 feet from a scaffold. He is unconscious and brought in on a spinal board. You wish to 'log roll' him off the spinal board. Which single instruction to the team about a log roll should be given? ★

A A rectal examination must be performed first

B Five members of staff are required in total

C One staff member should take the patient's shoulders and pelvis

D The patient's head must be held slightly flexed on the body

E The staff member who examines the patient's back is in charge

12. A 23-year-old woman has been tackled during a football match and has a fracture of the tibial plateau, which is undisplaced. Which is the single most appropriate method of immobilizing this fracture? ★

A Above-knee back slab

B Below-knee back slab

C Cast brace

D Cricket bat splint

E Wool and crêpe bandage

13. A 2-year-old boy is brought to the Emergency Department from his nursery. The nursery staff are concerned because he has multiple bruises on his arms and legs. Which single injury is the most likely to be non-accidental? ★

A Bruising to the anterior shins

B Dislocation of the radial head (a 'pulled elbow')

C Greenstick fracture of the distal radius

D Hot water splash burns to the arm and face

E Small, round bruises on the sides of the chest

14. A 75-year-old man has an acutely red left eye and is vomiting. His visual acuity is 6/24 and he appears very unwell. The eye is red; the cornea is hazy, and the pupil is irregular and unreactive. Which is the single most likely diagnosis? ★

A Acute closed-angle glaucoma

B Central retinal vein thrombosis

C Conjunctivitis

D Episcleritis

E Herpetic ulcer

15. A 34-year-old man is crushed against a wall by a reversing car. He is distressed and has difficulty breathing. Which is the single most reliable sign of a right-sided tension pneumothorax? ★

A Absent breath sounds on the right side

B Dullness of the chest to percussion

C Hyper-resonance to percussion

D The presence of circulatory shock

E Tracheal deviation to the left

16. A 25-year-old man has had a generalized seizure that lasted for 5 minutes. He remains post-ictal and his breathing is noisy. Which single piece of equipment is the most appropriate to use to maintain a patent airway? ★

A Endotracheal tube

B Guedel airway

C Nasopharyngeal airway

D Suction

E Tracheostomy tube

17. A 6-week-old boy has been vomiting immediately after every feed for the last 5 days. He vomits large quantities of non-bilious vomitus, which shoot out all over his mother while she is feeding him. He is screaming hungrily and has sunken eyes and dry mucous membranes. Which is the single most likely diagnosis? ★

A Hirschsprung's disease

B Malrotation of the bowel

C Oesophageal atresia

D Pyloric stenosis

E Urinary tract infection

18. A 54-year-old railway worker is hit by a train. He has an open injury to his right thigh, with a fractured femur clearly visible in the wound. There is arterial bleeding from the wound, and his systolic blood pressure is 70 mmHg. Which is the single most appropriate immediate action? ★

A Activate the major haemorrhage protocol

B Apply a tourniquet proximally

C Apply pressure to the wound

D Ask the surgeon to cross-clamp the femoral artery

E Explore the wound to clamp the bleeding vessel

19. A 35-year-old man has acute pain in his upper abdomen, radiating through to his back, and he is vomiting. Which single factor is most likely to support a diagnosis of pancreatitis? ★

A Contact with gastroenteritis

B Excessive alcohol intake

C History of foreign travel

D History of renal colic

E Use of cocaine and amphetamines

20. A 25-year-old woman has vaginal bleeding. Her husband tells you that they have been undergoing fertility treatment, and she is thought to be 2 months pregnant after implantation of fertilized eggs. She has some bleeding from her vagina, with mild left-sided abdominal tenderness. She has a pulse rate of 60 bpm and a systolic blood pressure of 80 mmHg. Which is the single most appropriate action to take in the Emergency Department? ★

A Arrange an urgent ultrasound scan of her pelvis

B Arrange for her to go to theatre

C Give her O-negative blood

D Give her O-positive blood

E Perform a speculum examination

21. A 41-year-old cyclist is brought into the Emergency Department after a collision with a motor vehicle. He appears pale and clammy. His blood pressure is 65/30 mmHg, and his heart rate is 145 bpm. He has a grossly hyper-expanded left hemithorax, with tracheal deviation to the right. The neck veins are visibly distended. Which is the single most appropriate initial management? ★

A Bolus 1 L of colloid

B Insert a chest drain

C Perform needle thoracocentesis

D Perform pericardiocentesis

E Transfuse 2 units of O-negative blood

22. A 45-year-old man presents with tachycardia, and the electro-cardiogram (ECG) is shown in Figure 13.1 (see Colour Plate section). Which single feature is an adverse sign in patients with this condition? ★★

A Abdominal pain

B Agitation and confusion

C Systolic blood pressure higher than 180 mmHg

D Redness of the extremities

E Basal crepitations and raised jugular venous pressure

23. A 25-year-old woman has taken 40 paracetamol tablets (20 g). She is refusing to accept medical treatment, stating that she wishes to die. Which is the single most appropriate immediate course of action? ★★

A Allow her to go home, as everyone has a right to die

B Assume that she is mentally incompetent and treat her against her wishes

C Contact her general practitioner (GP) for more information about her

D Formally assess her capacity to refuse treatment

E Request psychiatry to section her for medical treatment

24. A 95-year-old woman has a leg ulcer on the medial aspect of her lower leg. It is weeping, with necrotic tissue in the centre of the ulcer. After debridement under local anaesthesia, the wound looks pink and has some minor bleeding areas. Which is the single most appropriate dressing to apply? ★★

A Alginate dressing

B Flamazine cream

C Hydrocolloid dressing

D Iodine-impregnated dressing

E Non-adherent dressing

25. A 43-year-old woman is in a coma. To a painful stimulus, she opens her eyes, groans, and extends her arms. Which is her single Glasgow Coma Scale score? ★★

A 3

B 6

C 9

D 12

E 15

26. A 12-year-old boy presents to the Emergency Department 1 hour after clashing heads while playing football. Which single aspect of his presentation warrants computed tomography (CT) imaging of his head? ★ ★

A He has vomited twice in the Emergency Department

B He has a Glasgow Coma Scale (GCS) score of 14

C He has had a seizure in the Emergency Department

D He is bleeding profusely from a forehead laceration

E He reports a pain score of 10/10

27. A 22-year-old male student presents to the Emergency Department after a long train journey. He has noticed non-specific chest pain for the last hour and wanted to get it checked out. He is a non-smoker who is normally well and has no previous medical or significant family history. The electrocardiogram (ECG) is normal. Which single blood test would be useful in this situation? ★ ★

A Coagulation screen

B C-reactive protein

C D-dimer

D Serum amylase

E Troponin T

28. A 68-year-old man is pronounced dead in the Emergency Department after prolonged resuscitation. Which single factor in the history below requires reporting of the death to the coroner/procurator fiscal? ★ ★ ★

A The death is related to a diagnosed terminal illness

B The death is related to travel overseas

C The patient had been in hospital for less than 24 hours

D The patient fell and hit his head earlier in the day.

E The patient is not a UK citizen

29. You are walking home from work as a foundation doctor near the railway line when you hear a massive noise. A mainline train has derailed and is lying on its side. There appear to be multiple casualties. Which is the single most appropriate action? ★ ★ ★

A Make your way to the nearest hospital to offer help

B Provide immediate first aid to the nearest casualty

C Telephone 999 and give a formal report

D Telephone the press to give them the news

E Telephone your hospital to let them know

30. An 18-year-old man has been fitting for the last 15 minutes. An oxygen mask is in place and a nasal airway has been inserted by the ambulance crew. One dose of rectal diazepam has been given and a cannula has been inserted. Which is the single most appropriate immediate treatment? ★ ★ ★

A Diazepam 10 mg per rectum

B Lorazepam 4 mg intravenously (IV)

C Midazolam 4 mg IV

D Phenytoin 18 mg/kg IV

E Thiopentone 5 mg/kg IV

31. A 75-year-old diabetic woman has a pre-tibial laceration to her right leg that she sustained 45 minutes ago. She has a barely palpable popliteal pulse and no pulses in the foot. Which is the single most appropriate method of closure? ★ ★ ★ ★

A 30 Ethibond (semi-synthetic) sutures

B 40 Vicryl Rapide sutures

C Primary skin grafting

D Steri-strips

E Tissue glue

32. A 72-year-old man is acutely short of breath and unwell; his oxygen saturation on air is 75%, and his blood gases show a mildly raised carbon dioxide level and a low oxygen level with a mild mixed acidosis. Which single factor is a contraindication to the use of non-invasive ventilation (NIV) in this patient? ★ ★ ★ ★

A Epistaxis

B False teeth

C Nausea

D Pneumonia

E Previous respiratory arrest

33. A 75-year-old man has collapsed. He has left-sided facial weakness and a dense left hemiparesis. He is looking towards his right side and appears to have left-sided neglect. There is no obvious visual field deficit. He has severe dysarthria, but no obvious dysphasia. The computed tomography (CT) brain scan performed at 6 hours is suggestive of an ischaemic area in the distribution of the right middle cerebral artery. Which single intervention is most likely to optimize his outcome? ★ ★ ★ ★

A Keep his heart rate between 60 and 100 bpm

B Keep his temperature above 37.5°C

C Keep his systolic blood pressure below 100 mmHg

D Maintain his blood glucose level within the normal range

E Maintain his haemoglobin level above 12 g/dL

34. A 78-year-old man is in shock. After initial resuscitation, the decision is made to insert a central line using the subclavian approach. Which is the single most appropriate landmark to give guidance during the procedure? ★ ★ ★ ★

A Insertion is at the junction of the medial and middle thirds of the clavicle

B The clavicle is superior to the subclavian vein

C The needle should be pointing towards the tip of the contralateral scapula

D The subclavian vein lies medial to the subclavian artery

E The subclavian vein runs under the first rib

35. You are asked to act as team leader during the resuscitation of a 30-year-old man. Which is the single most effective behaviour of a team leader? ★ ★ ★ ★

A Check the identity and skills of all team members when they arrive

B Continually ask team members for their opinion

C Insist on silence during the resuscitation unless questioned directly

D Issue all instructions in a loud voice

E Personally perform all invasive procedures

ANSWERS

1. D ★   OHCS 10th edn → p. 753

In any major trauma, it is important to consider the possibility of a cervical spine injury. Current guidelines recommend full cervical spine immobilization in patients in whom an injury is suspected. Full protection consists of three-point immobilization using a correctly sized semi-rigid cervical collar, blocks to both sides of the head, and tape. Manual in-line immobilization should be used until these are available.

→ http://www.nice.org.uk/guidance/ng41/chapter/Recommendations (National Institute for Health and Care Excellence (2016). *Spinal injury: assessment and early management*. NICE guideline, NG41)

2. A ★

This woman has a markedly raised blood sugar level and is acidotic, which indicates diabetic ketoacidosis. After control of airway and breathing, which should always come first, the next priority is to restore circulating volume with a fluid bolus. Crystalloids are recommended for resuscitation, and sodium chloride 0.9% is the most commonly used. Potassium is only replaced once the patient has an adequate blood pressure and the serum potassium level is less than 5.5 mmol/L. Insulin should be given by a fixed-rate intravenous infusion, started at 0.1 U/kg/hour, once fluid resuscitation has commenced.

→ http://www.diabetes.org.uk/Documents/About%20Us/What%20 we%20say/Management-of-DKA-241013.pdf (Joint British Diabetes Societies Inpatient Care Group guideline (2013). *The management of diabetic ketoacidosis in adults*.)

3. C ★   OHCS 10th edn → p. 632

Lidocaine is the anaesthetic of choice, and 1–2 mL of 1% lidocaine is sufficient for the majority of wounds. Ring blocks essentially use infiltration of a local anaesthetic into the soft tissue around the digital nerve. This results in nerve impulses being blocked before they reach the spinal cord and cerebral cortex, thus achieving anaesthesia. Two injections are required, one on each side of the finger at the base of the finger. The whole skin of the finger will be anaesthetized by such a block, including the nail bed. There is no greater advantage of 2% lidocaine over 1%, and Emergency Departments are recommended to keep only one strength in stock, in order to minimize the risk of confusion when calculating doses. Although prilocaine and bupivacaine could theoretically be used, their much longer onset time makes them impractical for performing wound repairs in the Emergency Department. The use of adrenaline (epinephrine) in any local infiltration around an end artery (the digital artery) is contraindicated because of the risk of perfusion to the distal finger. Other end arteries include the nasal artery and the artery to the penis. The following websites describe how to perform a digital nerve block.

→ http://www.ncemi.org/cse/cse1011.htm
→ http://www.nysora.com/techniques/nerve-stimulator-and-surface-
based-ra-techniques/upper-extremitya/3023-digital-nerve-block.html

4. D ★   OHCS 10th edn → p. 544

This patient is most likely to have developed otitis media in association
with her viral upper respiratory tract infection, which has led to perforation of her eardrum and discharge of pus. It is unlikely that her symptoms are due to a simple otitis externa, as this rarely gives systemic
symptoms such as fever in an adult. Although a foreign body may act
as a nidus for infection, it is unlikely that the woman's earpiece would
have migrated into her ear without being noticed. Wax should not cause
systemic upset. An isolated perforation of the eardrum should not cause
continued discharge or temperature.

5. C ★   OHCS 10th edn → p. 726

The objective of immobilization must be considered. This fracture is
undisplaced, and as there are no strong forces working across the fracture site to cause displacement, it will heal well in time; therefore, the
key aim of immobilization is pain relief. A collar and cuff is the most
appropriate form of immobilization. It provides the support needed
without being too restrictive and allows early mobilization, which has
been suggested to improve long-term function. Some clinicians use a
broad arm sling, but this conveys no advantage and is generally more
restrictive.

A high arm sling flexes the elbow to over 90° and is therefore uncom-
fortable in the presence of an elbow effusion. A Futura splint (a remov-
able splint that immobilizes the wrist) is not appropriate for the elbow.
Complete immobilization of the elbow is unnecessary, making a back
slab unsuitable.

6. D ★

Erythromycin can inhibit the metabolism of warfarin by affecting the
cytochrome P450 complex in the liver, and it can therefore enhance its
effects. Aspirin and clopidogrel are both antiplatelet agents and could
increase the risk of bleeding. However, they would not affect the INR.

7. E ★

This is quite common in the elderly, and consideration should be given to
ensuring that it does not keep happening. Occupational therapy services
can assess the home environment and daily functioning and can address
issues that may predispose to falls.

8. E ★

This patient is having an upper gastrointestinal bleed and is showing clinical
evidence of haemorrhagic shock. The clinical priority in the Emergency

Department is fluid resuscitation in order to restore the circulating volume. In this case, the most appropriate fluid to use is blood, and this should be given in line with departmental transfusion/major haemorrhage policies. Many Emergency Departments have their own blood fridges. However, if blood is not immediately available, then giving a balanced crystalloid (e.g Hartmann's solution) would be suitable as a short-term measure. Colloids generally do not convey any benefit over crystalloids in this situation; they are more expensive, and there is some limited evidence that they may be associated with increased morbidity and mortality.

→ http://www.transfusionguidelines.org.uk

→ http://www.nice.org.uk/guidance/CG174/chapter/1-Recommendations (National Institute for Health and Care Excellence (2013). *Intravenous fluid therapy in adults in hospital.* Clinical guideline CG74)

→ http://www.cochrane.org/CD000567/INJ_are-colloids-more-effective-than-crystalloids-in-reducing-death-in-people-who-are-critically-ill-or-injured (Perel P, Roberts I, Ker K (2013). *Are colloids more effective than crystalloids in reducing death in people who are critically ill or injured?* Cochrane review)

9. A ★

The sudden onset of severe occipital headache suggests a subarachnoid haemorrhage. All of these symptoms may occur in a patient with a subarachnoid haemorrhage, but loss of consciousness suggests rising intracranial pressure and must be treated as an emergency.

10. B ★

This man is significantly shocked and requires fluid resuscitation. A large-bore line is needed in order to provide rapid fluid administration, and a 14G cannula is the most appropriate device to deliver this. Central lines are generally not used for fluid resuscitation, as fluids cannot be given as rapidly down them (due to the length of the line) and they take longer to insert. The use of intraosseous needles in adults is becoming increasingly common, and they are a good alternative if venous access cannot be achieved quickly. However, they should not be the device of choice.

11. B ★   OHCS 10th edn → p. 782

Five people are required to perform a log roll. One person stands at the patient's head and keeps control of the head, neck, and airway and gives commands; one takes the arms and trunk; one takes the upper legs and pelvis; one supports the calves, and the fifth person examines the back and performs a rectal examination. The patient is rolled gently towards the three supporters of the body and then held in a stable line while the back is examined.

12. A ★   OHCS 10th edn → p. 735

The most important issue in this fracture is to consider what is attached to the fracture site, and therefore what the possible displacement or consequences of not immobilizing might be. The tibial plateau is a weight-bearing surface, so any fracture must be treated as non-weight-bearing at first. In addition, the injury pattern often includes injuries to the menisci or collateral ligaments. If the fracture involves the cruciate ligaments (evidenced by involvement of the tibial spine in the fracture line), minimizing the anteroposterior movement of the tibia on the femur is important. Immobilization techniques must be easy for the patient to manage and maintain their mobility. Therefore, the most appropriate technique for immobilization in the Emergency Department is the above-knee back slab. A below-knee back slab will not restrict the anteroposterior movement of the tibia on the femur. The cast brace is more suitable once the patient has started to mobilize the knee after the initial injury has settled. A cricket bat splint may be useful, as it will allow the patient to wash their leg, but may not be available in the Emergency Department. A wool and crêpe bandage was formerly a useful method but is no longer used because of the extensive resources required and the difficulty for the patient in keeping such a bandage correctly applied.

13. E ★   OHCS 10th edn → p. 146

Accidents are common in toddlers, and it can be hard to work out which of them are non-accidental. The shins are a very common site for bruising, but the chest, abdomen, and back are not. Small discrete round bruises suggest the use of fingers or an implement. Pulled elbows and greenstick fractures are common in young children, and burns that have splash patterns are more commonly accidental.

→ http://www.nice.org.uk/guidance/cg89 (National Institute for Health and Care Excellence (2009). *Child maltreatment: when to suspect maltreatment in under 18s*. Clinical guideline CG89)

→ https://cks.nice.org.uk/child-maltreatment-recognition-and-management (National Institute for Health and Care Excellence (2014). *Child maltreatment—recognition and management*. Clinical Knowledge Summaries)

14. A ★   OHCS 10th edn → p. 433

This is an ophthalmological emergency, caused by blockage of the flow of the aqueous humour from the anterior chamber, which is exacerbated at night when the pupil dilates. It leads to raised intraocular pressure, which causes severe pain, redness, a fixed pupil, and decreased acuity. Drops are required to cause miosis and open the angle.

15. D ★   OHCS 10th edn → p. 788

Tension pneumothorax is an emergency and should be looked for as part of the primary survey in trauma patients, although spotting it is not always easy. If a patient is in respiratory distress, the most reliable sign that a tension pneumothorax is present is the evidence of haemodynamic compromise due to compression and displacement of the mediastinum, restricting venous return to the heart. Reduced breath sounds could be due to a variety of reasons and do not necessarily indicate a tension pneumothorax. Other signs are tracheal deviation to the opposite side and hyper-resonance to percussion, but these are unreliable signs and can be difficult to elicit. Other causes of circulatory shock in a trauma patient must also be considered.

16. C ★

Patients who are post-ictal may need airway support until they become fully conscious. Guedel (oropharyngeal) airways and suction may trigger a gag reflex. Nasopharyngeal airways are generally well tolerated. Intubation may be necessary if the patient does not regain full consciousness within a reasonable time frame or if there is further airway compromise for any other reason.

17. D ★   OHCS 10th edn → p. 172

This child has a classic presentation of pyloric stenosis. It typically presents at 6–8 weeks with projectile milky vomits during or immediately after feeds. There is constipation and the baby seems to be hungry all the time, as he has had no food. A mass may be felt in the midline during a feed and peristalsis may be seen, but the only reliable way to diagnose pyloric stenosis is with an ultrasound scan.

18. C ★   OHCS 10th edn → pp. 781, 784

Haemorrhage control is part of the assessment and initial management of circulation. This should be done by applying direct pressure on bleeding points in the first instance. If this failed to control the bleeding, then applying a tourniquet may be an appropriate measure. Activating the major haemorrhage pathway should be done, along with the above measures, in cases where bleeding is ongoing and the patient is haemodynamically compromised. However, the initial priority should be to control the bleeding.

19. B ★

This is the most likely cause of pancreatitis in a young man. Excess alcohol consumption, both in the form of binge drinking and long-term increased consumption, can cause acute pancreatitis. Some other causes of pancreatitis include gallstones, abdominal trauma, post-endoscopic retrograde cholangiopancreatography (ERCP), steroid use, antibiotics, hyperlipidaemia, and the commonly remembered (but never seen) scorpion venom!

20. E ★   OHCS 10th edn → p. 260

In a miscarriage, products of conception can build up behind the cervical os and cause pressure. The cervix has many stretch receptors, and when it is trying to dilate, it can stimulate the vagus nerve, causing haemodynamic instability. This causes bradycardia because of the vagal stimulation, rather than the tachycardia that is seen in severe blood loss. A speculum examination needs to be performed and these products removed under direct vision with sponge forceps, which may result in an improvement in haemodynamic status. Fluid resuscitation and further surgical treatment may be needed if the blood pressure remains low. An ultrasound scan should be performed to assess the pregnancy, but the haemodynamic instability here (as evidenced by a *relative* bradycardia) makes other options more urgent.

→ https://www.nice.org.uk/guidance/cg154 (National Institute for Health and Care Excellence (2012). *Ectopic pregnancy and miscarriage: diagnosis and initial management.* Clinical guideline CG154)

21. C ★   OHCS 10th edn → p. 788

This is a classic presentation of a tension pneumothorax. This life-threatening condition requires immediate needle thoracocentesis, i.e. insertion of a wide-bore cannula into the pleural cavity, followed by chest drain insertion.

→ http://lifeinthefastlane.com/ccc/emergency-thoracocentesis/

22. E ★★

This is a broad-complex tachycardia. If the patient is stable, it can be treated with drugs, most commonly amiodarone. However, in a patient with adverse signs (chest pain, signs of heart failure, or shock), electrical cardioversion should be performed.

→ https://www.resus.org.uk/resuscitation-guidelines/peri-arrest-arrhythmias/#tachy (Advanced Life Support tachycardia algorithm)

23. D ★★   OHCS 10th edn → p. 409

The Mental Capacity Act 2005 (England and Wales) states that everyone should be treated as being able to make their own decisions until it has been shown that they cannot. It also aims to enable people to make their own decisions for as long as they are capable of doing so. In order to have capacity, an individual must be able to understand the information being given to them, to retain and weigh up this information, and to communicate their decision. A lack of capacity could be permanent or temporary, and an individual's capacity to make a decision must be established at the time when a decision needs to be made. A lack of capacity could be due to a severe learning disability, dementia, mental health problems, a brain injury, a stroke, or unconsciousness due to an anaesthetic or a sudden accident. Note that a different Act—the Adults with Incapacity (Scotland) Act 2000—applies in Scotland.

→ http://www.nhs.uk/Conditions/social-care-and-support-guide/Pages/mental-capacity.aspx

→ http://www.scie.org.uk/mca/introduction/mental-capacity-act-2005-at-a-glance

→ http://www.legislation.gov.uk/ukpga/2005/9/contents

24. E ★★

A non-adherent dressing is recommended after debridement. Iodine-impregnated dressings may cause local inflammation and reaction, and are not to be recommended. Alginate dressings have advantages, particularly when the wound has a heavy exudate, but immediately after debridement, these should not be necessary. Hydrocolloid dressings can be used, but they have not been shown to have any benefit over a simple non-adherent dressing.

→ https://cks.nice.org.uk/leg-ulcer-venous#!scenario

25. B ★   OHCS 10th edn → p. 778

The Glasgow Coma Scale score is calculated, as shown in Table 9.2.

26. C ★★   OHCS 10th edn → pp. 790–1

The National Institute for Health and Care Excellence (NICE) guidelines on the management of head injury state that if a post-traumatic seizure occurs, CT imaging of the head is indicated. As this patient is a child, he would need to vomit three times before a scan was indicated, but a single vomit in an adult following a head injury would prompt CT scanning. In a child, a GCS score of 14 on presentation is not an indication for a CT head. However, if the GCS score remains less than 15 after 2 hours, a CT scan would be indicated at this point.

→ https://www.nice.org.uk/guidance/cg176/chapter/1-Recommendations (National Institute for Health and Care Excellence (2014). *Head injury: assessment and early management*. Clinical guideline CG176)

27. C ★★

The D-dimer blood test is only useful if the result is normal, because it can then be used to rule out venous thromboembolism in low-risk patients. D-dimer is a fibrin degradation product which indicates that clotting and subsequent fibrinolysis have been occurring. It is therefore non-specific and will be raised in many situations (e.g. post-operatively). Local protocols may recommend it in a situation where clinical suspicion of pulmonary embolism (based on risk factors and clinical presentation) is low. The D-dimer test can be performed to enable discharge of the patient with more confidence.

Troponin T is only indicated if there is a suspicion that chest pain may have an ischaemic aetiology. There is nothing to suggest this in this case. The other tests have no role in managing this presentation.

28. D ★★★

It is important to know which deaths need to be reported to the coroner/procurator fiscal. Deaths that may be due to an accident should always be reported, even if the cause of death is known. It used to be the case that all deaths occurring within 24 hours of admission had to be reported. However, in 2016, the chief coroner advised that this was no longer necessary, provided a cause of death could be given. The following website provides guidance.

→ https://www.gov.uk/after-a-death/when-a-death-is-reported-to-a-coroner

29. C ★★★   OHCS 10th edn → p. 813

Although it may be tempting to help out at major incidents, these are carefully controlled and managed by trained personnel, and your responsibility, even as a doctor, is to allow these teams to take charge and to act as any other member of the public, unless specifically instructed to do otherwise. Your hospital will have a major incident plan, and they will contact you directly if your help is needed.

30. B ★★★

There are well-established treatment algorithms for the management of status epilepticus. The first-line treatment consists of benzodiazepines. Diazepam is administered per rectum if there is no IV access, but lorazepam is preferred once IV access has been established. Phenytoin and thiopentone may be required, but only if the patient has failed to respond to the use of IV benzodiazepines.

→ http://www.patient.co.uk/showdoc/40001332

→ https://www.nice.org.uk/guidance/cg137/chapter/appendix-f-protocols-for-treating-convulsive-status-epilepticus-in-adults-and-children-adults-published-in-2004-and-children-published-in-2011 (National Institute for Health and Care Excellence (2012). *Epilepsies: diagnosis and management*. Clinical guideline CG137—protocol for treating convulsive status epilepticus in adults and children)

31. D ★★★★   OHCS 10th edn → pp. 772–3

Pre-tibial lacerations are difficult to heal, even when there is no coexisting morbidity. In this patient with both major vessel arterial disease and probable microvascular disease, the blood supply will be severely limited. Any attempt at closure must ensure that the edges are approximated as closely as possible but are not under excessive tension, that there are no foreign bodies in the wound, and that the flap itself is cleaned as thoroughly as possible. Steri-strips under as little tension as possible are the most appropriate method of skin closure in this patient. Some minor 'spot welds' of glue might also help to minimize tension, while still allowing exudate to leave the wound.

Vicryl Rapide is a dissolving suture (after 7–10 days) that is suitable for subcutaneous sutures, but it is not appropriate for this wound as the healing time may be up to 6 weeks. Ethibond can be used to close wounds but would be too heavy and would lead to tissue strangulation between the sutures. Although a proportion of pre-tibial lacerations result in skin grafting, primary grafting is not recommended because of the risk associated with anaesthetic and the creation of a second wound, particularly in a high-risk patient such as this diabetic woman with arteriopathy.

→ https://cks.nice.org.uk/lacerations

32. **A** ★★★★

NIV is a method of respiratory support used to reduce the work of breathing and improve ventilation in patients with type 2 respiratory failure. If used in the correct patients, it can prevent the need for invasive ventilation and the complications associated with this. Patients receive positive pressure ventilation via a tight-fitting facial mask or specialist high-flow nasal cannulae. NIV is contraindicated in patients who are unable to wear the mask due to facial trauma or burns, are actively vomiting or have epistaxis, have a reduced conscious level, are unable to protect their airway, or have an untreated pneumothorax. Well-fitting dentures can be left in, as this helps to maintain the facial structure and promotes a good seal with the mask. However, if they are poorly fitting, then they should be removed. A previous respiratory arrest does not prevent the use of NIV. However, it does suggest that it may not be successful and the patient should be monitored closely and the treatment escalated early if appropriate.

→ https://www.brit-thoracic.org.uk/document-library/clinical-information/acute-hypercapnic-respiratory-failure/bts-guidelines-for-ventilatory-management-of-ahrf/ (British Thoracic Society (2016). *Guidelines for the ventilatory management of acute hypercapnic respiratory failure in adults.*)

→ http://lifeinthefastlane.com/ccc/non-invasive-ventilation-niv/

33. **D** ★★★★

Hyperglycaemia after stroke worsens brain injury. Large randomized controlled trials have shown that keeping blood sugar levels within tight limits leads to better outcomes. Current guidelines advise maintaining a blood sugar level between 4 and 11 mmol/L. Hypotension should be prevented in order to maintain cerebral perfusion and where possible normothermia should be maintained, as pyrexia has been shown to be associated with a worse outcome.

→ Gentile NT, Seftchick MW, Huynh T, Kruus LK, Gaughan J. Decreased mortality by normalising blood glucose after acute ischemic stroke. *Acad Emerg Med.* 2006;**13**:174–80.

→ https://www.nice.org.uk/guidance/cg68/chapter/1-Guidance (National Institute for Health and Care Excellence (2008). *Stroke and transient ischaemic attack in over 16s: diagnosis and initial management.* Clinical guideline CG68)

34. **B** ★★★★

The safest method of obtaining central venous access is to do it under ultrasound guidance, as this improves the chances of successful venous cannulation and reduces complications. However, in some circumstances, this may not be possible, and therefore a landmark technique can be used.

→ http://www.anaesthesiauk.com/SearchRender.aspx?DocId=1406&I
ndex=D%3a%5cdtSearch%5cUserData%5cAUK&HitCount=3&hits=3
+e+125+

35. A ★★★★

Being an effective team leader is a skill which requires practice, just like any other. In order to lead a team effectively, it is important to know your team members and their skill set. In medicine, a team can often be working together for the first time, and so checking these things when the team members arrive is essential. The team leader should ideally remain 'hands-off' in order to maintain an overview of the resuscitation.

Chapter 14

Pre-hospital care

Oliver Harrison

Many doctors are attracted to pre-hospital emergency medicine (PHEM) because of the variety of challenges that it presents. With limited time and resources, the doctor is expected to assess and treat a range of medical and traumatic pathologies in patients of any age, without delaying transport to the most appropriate location for definitive care. This must be done in spite of what is usually a suboptimal environment, e.g. in a ditch at the roadside, on a rainy building site, or in a crowded town centre. Recognizing the limitations of what can be achieved on scene is a key skill that must be balanced against the increasing range of lifesaving interventions at the disposal of pre-hospital teams.

While PHEM has been practised by a variety of doctors for many years, it has only recently gained General Medical Council (GMC) subspecialty recognition. A formal training programme may now be undertaken by trainees with base specialties of acute medicine, anaesthetics, emergency medicine, and intensive care medicine, leading to a dual certificate of completion of training. The challenging nature of the pre-hospital environment, the high-risk nature of the interventions that can be undertaken, and the lack of availability of immediate assistance on scene mean that PHEM is a service delivered by consultants and senior trainees. Medical students and foundation doctors who may be interested in PHEM training should seek to spend time in the above mentioned acute specialties, as well as looking for opportunities to observe alongside some of the services that operate nationally.

The following questions represent a small selection of the range of scenarios that may be faced by a PHEM practitioner on a day-to-day basis.

QUESTIONS

1. Pre-hospital responders attend a 40-year-old female who is known to have a history of asthma. She is unable to complete full sentences, has a respiratory rate of 30 breaths/minute, a pulse rate of 122 bpm, and an oxygen saturation of 95% on air. Which is the single most appropriate initial management for this patient in the pre-hospital environment? ★

A Administer 5 mg nebulized salbutamol, 500 micrograms nebulized ipratropium bromide, and 10 mg intravenous (IV) hydrocortisone, and transport to the Emergency Department

B Administer 5 mg nebulized salbutamol using an air-driven nebulizer, and transport to the Emergency Department

C Administer salbutamol via a metered-dose inhaler and spacer device, and transport to the Emergency Department

D Administer salbutamol via a metered-dose inhaler and spacer device until symptoms improve, then advise follow-up by the patient's general practitioner (GP)

E Rapid sequence induction of anaesthesia, mechanical ventilation, and transfer to the nearest Intensive Care Unit.

2. A 68-year-old male suffers a cardiac arrest in a public place. Following arrival of the emergency services, the patient is found to be in ventricular fibrillation. The third shock is about to be given. Which is the single most appropriate action after delivery of the third shock? ★ ★ ★

A Administer 1 mg adrenaline (epinephrine) and 300 mg amiodarone

B Administer 10 mL 1:10 000 adrenaline (epinephrine)

C Continue cardiopulmonary resuscitation (CPR) for a further 2 minutes before checking for a pulse

D Continue CPR while another responder assesses cardiac activity using subcostal ultrasound

E Pause CPR and check for a pulse

3. A lady who is 36 weeks pregnant delivers her baby unexpectedly at home. On arrival of the emergency services, the baby is found to be floppy, centrally cyanosed, and taking occasional gasps despite being dried and stimulated. Which is the single most appropriate next step in the treatment of the baby? ★ ★ ★

A Commence cardiopulmonary resuscitation (CPR) at a ratio of three compressions to one breath

B Commence CPR at a ratio of 15 compressions to two breaths

C Deliver five inflation breaths using a bag–valve–mask connected to air

D Deliver five inflation breaths using a bag–valve–mask connected to oxygen

E Intubate the baby and ventilate at a rate of 30–40 breaths/minute

4. A male in his 50s is extricated from a house fire. On initial assessment, he displays no signs of airway or breathing compromise, but both his legs appear to have significant burns. Which is the single best initial step in managing this patient? ★ ★ ★

A Apply cling film to all burnt areas, avoiding circumferential wrapping

B Apply water gel dressings to all burnt areas

C Clearly document the extent of full-thickness and partial-thickness burns before applying dressings

D Cool the burns under running water for 20 minutes

E Gain intravenous (IV) access, and administer 0.9% sodium chloride in a volume determined by the Parkland formula

5. A 32-year-old tree surgeon sustains a chainsaw injury to his right anterior thigh. There is significant blood loss from the wound, and the patient is complaining of severe pain. Which is the single most appropriate first step in managing this patient in the pre-hospital environment? ★ ★ ★

A Apply a Combat Application Tourniquet proximal to the area of bleeding, and tighten until haemorrhage stops

B Apply oxygen, and examine the chest before addressing the bleeding

C Gain intravenous (IV) access in order to administer tranexamic acid and analgesia

D Lie the patient supine, apply direct pressure to the wound, and elevate the limb

E Pack the wound with Celox gauze

6. An 11-year-old child who is known to have a peanut allergy develops severe shortness of breath and wheeze while having lunch at school. On arrival of the ambulance crew, the child has oedema of the mouth and appears cyanosed. Which is the single best dose and route of adrenaline (epinephrine) to administer to this child? ★★★

A 300 micrograms intramuscularly

B 500 micrograms intramuscularly

C 300 micrograms intravenously

D 500 micrograms intravenously

E 150 micrograms intravenously

7. A 15-year-old male has sustained a stab injury to the epigastrium with a knife of unknown length. On arrival of the emergency services, he is pale, clammy, and agitated. He has a pulse rate of 128 bpm, a blood pressure of 88/48 mmHg, and a respiratory rate of 34 breaths/minute. Air entry is present and equal bilaterally on auscultation. Which is the single most likely diagnosis? ★★★

A Cardiac tamponade

B Flail chest

C Massive haemothorax

D Simple pneumothorax

E Tension pneumothorax

8. A 65-year-old male patient is extricated from a car by the fire service, following a high-speed road traffic collision. He is suspected of having rib fractures and a humeral fracture and is complaining of tingling in his legs. His Glasgow Coma Scale (GCS) score is 15. To maintain in-line immobilization of the spine, he is transferred onto a long spinal board after removal of the car's roof. Which is the single best way of preparing this patient for onward transport to hospital? ★★★★

A Leave the patient on the long spinal board, and apply a cervical collar, blocks, and tape

B Leave the patient on the long spinal board without further immobilization

C Log roll the patient, and assess for spinal tenderness. If none is present, allow him to get up and lie directly on the ambulance stretcher

D Move the patient to the ambulance stretcher, then log roll to remove the spinal board. Apply a cervical collar, blocks, and tape

E Remove the patient from the spinal board using a scoop stretcher, and transport to hospital on this after applying a cervical collar, blocks, and tape

9. A 25-year-old motorcyclist is attended to by emergency services, having been hit by a car at 30 mph. He is complaining of severe pain to his mid-left thigh, which appears swollen. A closed fracture of the femoral shaft is suspected. Which is the single most appropriate way of managing this injury? ★ ★ ★ ★

A A long box splint to enclose the left lower limb

B Neighbour strapping to the adjacent limb

C No splint required as the fracture appears not to be displaced

D The Kendrick traction device (KTD)

E The SAM pelvic sling

10. Reports are received of an incident developing in a local shopping centre. A number of people have become incapacitated and others are complaining of symptoms, including watery eyes, blurred vision, difficulty breathing, and vomiting. Which is the single most likely chemical agent to have caused these symptoms? ★ ★ ★ ★

A Chlorine

B Cyanide

C Methane

D Phosgene

E Sarin

11. Emergency responders attend a local industrial unit, following reports of a collapsed, unconscious patient. On arrival, the responders notice through a window three patients lying apparently motionless on the floor. Which is the single best course of action for the attending crew? ★ ★ ★ ★

A Cautiously approach the scene, but retreat if any unusual odours are detected or gas clouds seen

B Drag the patients to a central location, so that sequential ABC assessments can be completed and all patients can be monitored

C Remain at a distance from the scene, prevent bystanders from gaining access, and pass a METHANE report to control

D Request backup from the Hazardous Area Response Team (HART)

E Request immediate backup of two further ambulances before proceeding to prioritize patients using the triage sieve system

12. A 32-year-old male weighing approximately 80 kg falls from the roof of his house and lands on the patio. An enhanced care team attends and finds him to have a suspected left-sided femoral fracture, rib fractures, and a boggy swelling to his temporal region. His pulse rate is 115 bpm, blood pressure 90/54 mmHg, and Glasgow Coma Scale (GCS) score E1 V2 M4 (7). The team decides to perform rapid sequence induction of anaesthesia due to his low GCS score. Which is the single best drug and dose to use for induction of anaesthesia in this patient? ★ ★ ★ ★

A Etomidate 25 mg

B Ketamine 80 mg

C Midazolam 16 mg

D Propofol 80 mg

E Thiopentone 400 mg

13. An intercity train derails, causing multiple casualties. Representatives from the three main emergency services gather at a remote location to develop the plans and coordinate the assets required to respond to the major incident. Which is the single most accurate phrase used to describe this group? ★ ★ ★ ★

A Gold coordination group

B Operational coordination group

C Silver coordination group

D Strategic coordination group

E Tactical coordination group

14. A 52-year-old motorcyclist hits the side of a car head on at 40 mph. On arrival of the emergency services, he is complaining of severe lower back pain. His pulse rate is 105 bpm and blood pressure 102/65 mmHg. He is wearing a full set of motorcycle leathers. Which is the single correct way of applying the pelvic binder on this patient? ★ ★ ★ ★

A At the level of the anterior superior iliac spines, following removal of the patient's clothing

B At the level of the greater trochanters, following removal of the patient's clothing

C At the level of the greater trochanters, over the top of the patient's clothing

D Just below the anterior superior iliac spines, following removal of the patient's clothing

E Just below the anterior superior lilac spines, over the top of the patient's clothing

15. An elderly male is found collapsed outside on a winter's night. He is unconscious, hypotensive, and bradycardic. His core temperature is measured as 31°C. A 12-lead electrocardiogram (ECG) is performed which shows an abnormality. Which is the single most likely ECG abnormality to be associated with hypothermia of this degree? ★ ★ ★ ★

A Delta waves

B J-waves

C P pulmonale

D Third-degree heart block

E U-waves

ANSWERS

1. A ★

This patient fulfils the criteria for acute severe asthma. First-line therapy includes β2-agonists, ipratropium, and steroids. Assessment in hospital is needed in case she develops life-threatening or near-fatal asthma.

→ https://www.brit-thoracic.org.uk/document-library/clinical-information/asthma/btssign-asthma-guideline-2016/

2. A ★★★

The Advanced Life Support algorithm for shockable rhythms states that 300 mg amiodarone should be given after the third shock, irrespective of whether the shocks have been consecutive or interrupted by CPR. Adrenaline should also be given after the third shock if it has not already been delivered for a non-shockable rhythm, in which case a dose should be given every 3–5 minutes. One milligram adrenaline is the dose contained in 10 mL of 1:10 000.

→ https://www.resus.org.uk/resuscitation-guidelines/

3. C ★★★   OHCS 10th edn → p. 107

If a newborn fails to breathe adequately after birth, the lungs remain filled with fluid and no oxygen is able to reach the heart. The priority is therefore to inflate the lungs—this is achieved by delivering inflation breaths of 2–3 seconds' duration, aiming to generate visible chest movement. In the majority of cases, this should lead to an increase in heart rate and commencement of spontaneous ventilation. If the heart rate fails to improve, CPR should be commenced using a 3:1 ratio.

→ https://www.resus.org.uk/resuscitation-guidelines/resuscitation-and-support-of-transition-of-babies-at-birth/

4. D ★★★   OHCS 10th edn → pp. 766–7

Cooling burns as soon as possible will stop the burning process, thus limiting the extent of injury. In order to achieve this, any burnt or burning clothes should be removed. Cooling burns will also have a significant analgesic effect. Once cooling has taken place, the burns can be dressed with cling film before transporting the patient to hospital. Accurate calculation of burn extent is difficult in the pre-hospital setting.

→ https://fphc.rcsed.ac.uk/media/1754/burns-patient-management.pdf

5. D ★★★   OHCS 10th edn → p. 781

A wound of this nature is likely to cause severe, if not catastrophic, haemorrhage due to the mechanism and location. Given that the patient is complaining of pain, it can be surmised that the airway is patent. Early control of the haemorrhage is paramount, and this should be carried out in a stepwise approach. This includes: direct pressure, bandaging (e.g. using the Oleas modular bandage), elevation above the level of the heart, packing with haemostatic gauze/granules (e.g. Celox), indirect pressure over a proximal artery, and finally application of a tourniquet if the haemorrhage is occurring from a limb. Blast injuries and traumatic amputations are likely to require immediate application of a tourniquet.

→ https://fphc.rcsed.ac.uk/media/1726/site-of-application-of-tourniquets.pdf

6. A ★★★ OHCS 10th edn → p. 237

The intramuscular route is preferred for administration of adrenaline in anaphylaxis. The use of intravenous adrenaline is only appropriate if the practitioner is experienced in its use and is aware of the appropriate dose to administer. Advanced Life Support guidelines state the dose of intramuscular adrenaline in a child 6–12 years old is 300 micrograms, or 0.3 mL of 1:1000.

→ https://www.resus.org.uk/anaphylaxis/emergency-treatment-of-anaphylactic-reactions/

7. A ★★★ OHCS 10th edn → p. 788

Penetrating injuries to the chest and epigastrium can easily result in injuries to the lungs and heart. This patient's rapid deterioration and lack of lateralizing signs suggest that cardiac tamponade is the most likely diagnosis. A massive haemothorax may result in similar haemodynamic changes, but these are unlikely to develop as quickly as when cardiac tamponade is the cause.

→ https://fphc.rcsed.ac.uk/media/1788/management-of-chest-injuries.pdf

8. E ★★★★

The long spinal board is an extrication device only—it should not be used for transport due to the risk of developing pressure sores. The scoop stretcher is recommended for use in transporting patients—it facilitates patient movement without needing repeated log rolls which are painful and risk disrupting internal clots.

→ https://fphc.rcsed.ac.uk/media/1766/minimal-patient-handling.pdf

9. D ★★★★ OHCS 10th edn → p. 811

The KTD is a portable, easily applied femoral traction splint. A particular advantage is that it can be used in the presence of a suspected or confirmed pelvic fracture. Splinting a suspected femoral fracture will reduce both pain and blood loss, by bringing the open bone ends together.

10. E ★★★★   OHCS 10th edn → p. 804

Sarin is a nerve agent that has previously been used in terrorist attacks. It is an acetylcholinesterase inhibitor that leads to parasympathetic symptoms and motor paralysis, including the respiratory muscles.

11. C ★★★★

The STEP 1-2-3-plus guidance describes the initial operational response to a potential chemical, biological, nuclear, radiological, or explosive incident. The presentation of three or more incapacitated casualties without explanation should prompt suspicion of such an incident and lead to the instigation of appropriate control measures and response escalation as soon as possible. Remaining at a distance from the scene prevents the responders from becoming victims of whatever has caused the casualties to become incapacitated.

12. B ★★★★

In haemodynamically unstable patients, an induction agent is required that does not cause a further drop in blood pressure. Unlike propofol or thiopentone, ketamine does not cause vasodilatation and also has sympathomimetic effects. Blood pressure is therefore less likely to be adversely affected by its administration. The normal dose is 2 mg/kg, but when patients are severely compromised, a reduced dose of 1 mg/kg should be used.

13. E ★★★★

According to the Joint Emergency Services Interoperability Programme, the three tiers of command are strategic, tactical, and operational. Previously, these tiers were known as gold, silver, and bronze, respectively. The tactical coordination group is concerned with developing the plans required to respond to an incident, while the operational teams on scene execute these plans.

→ http://www.jesip.org.uk/command

14. B ★★★★   OHCS 10th edn → p. 794

This patient has a mechanism and symptoms that would support the diagnosis of a pelvic injury, plus evidence of haemodynamic compromise. A pelvic binder should be placed next to the skin at the level of the greater trochanters. Placing over clothes puts the patient at risk of pressure injury and will necessitate removal of the binder at a later time to remove the clothing, thus potentially exacerbating the pelvic injury.

→ https://fphc.rcsed.ac.uk/media/1765/the-pre-hospital-management-of-pelvic-fractures.pdf

15. B ★★★★ OHCS 10th edn → p. 786

J-waves, or Osborne waves, are an extra positive deflection on the ECG, occurring just after the normal S-wave, at the J-point. They are commonest in leads II and V3–6. The height of the J-wave is approximately proportional to the degree of hypothermia. Atrial fibrillation is another ECG finding that is commonly seen in hypothermic patients.

Index

Note: Page numbers in *italics* denote answers